TAI CHI: THOUGHTS & THEORIES

An Exposition of the Tai Chi Classics

Dr. Frank Bisceglia EdD.

Copyright © 2020 Dr. Frank Bisceglia EdD.

All rights reserved

No part of this book may be reproduced, or stored in a retrieval system, or transmitted in any form or by any means, electronic, mechanical, photocopying, recording, or otherwise, without express written permission of the publisher.

CONTENTS

PREFACE

TAI CHI: THOUGHTS & THEORIES contains nothing new and is only a reminder of existing quotes, paraphrases, and suggestions from many sources, especially the Tai Chi Classics. Credit is given to the source, unless it's unknown. There are no secrets in Tai Chi, but there are several fundamental concepts that will enhance the attributes of Tai Chi, if implemented into one's practice and daily living. *TAI CHI: THOUGHTS & THEORIES* highlights many age-old adages in a simple and understandable format. These essays and notes are appropriate for any level of interest. Hopefully the comments and suggestions will encourage the reader to continue pursuing a more in-depth study and practice of Tai Chi.

***

Now that I'm in my 70's, I understand how Confucius felt in his senior years when he said "I wish I had another 50 years to study Tai Chi". As we age, we alter many of our personal filters that predispose how we interpret information. We are sometimes fortunate enough to see through the veil and perceive what is meant to be. As a result, I hope to share with others my interpretations of some of the most basic doctrines associated with Tai Chi. Using the essays from the Tai Chi Classics and several contemporary Masters, my intention is to emphasize some of the traditional techniques and clarify those that often appear to be incomprehensible, misleading, or dualistic.

***

For more than 1000 years Tai Chi was taught strictly by oral traditions. As various authors struggled to interpret and translate the fundamentals, many concepts were distorted, muddled, or deliberately deleted. In an attempt to convey the truth, some have devoted years to deliver an accurate translation. For example, Master Jyh-Jian Soong utilized 10 different translators over a 16-year period to convert the original Chinese version of his book *THE I CHIEN T'AI CHI CH'UAN* into an English edition.

***

The following thoughts and theories are based on documented quotes and erudite interpretations from various translations that have been used to illuminate the experiences associated with the study and practice of Tai Chi. This manual has been written in a clear and concise manner, based on scholarly knowledge and reliable resources.

***

This booklet highlights the significance of "Right Living" over superficial mechanics. This point is emphasized because many instructors, schools, and supplemental resources exaggerate the importance of proper techniques, while ignoring the core doctrine of spiritual growth.

***

The study of Tai Chi can best be explained as a complex puzzle involving various pieces that will take time, patience, and practice before grasping the many innuendos that accompany the true nature of this ancient art. As the age-old adage states, "You can't rush a caterpillar to evolve into a butterfly". Likewise, there are thoughts and theories we won't comprehend until we are ready for them.

***

Many of the concepts that make no sense in the early stages of study, will become more apparent with dedicated practice. Chuang-Tzu said this is known as "continuous transformation" (Chuang, 4th Century BC).

***

This booklet uses a format that repeats similar viewpoints by various Tai Chi Masters as a way to emphasize, clarify, and validate the concepts being presented. Also, many of the thoughts and theories are closely interrelated, so several of the same ideas are echoed throughout this exposition.

***

MANY PATHS

The purpose of this section is to soften any tone of pomposity or dogmatism that may unintentionally appear in the construct of this manual. The author is a firm believer that there are many Paths to reach the same end, and Tai Chi is only one of them.

***

Most of the thoughts and theories that define Tai Chi are only one way to obtain the physical, mental, and spiritual benefits associated with this unique style of gentle exercise.

***

Physically, you can get the same benefits from many other methods of exercise.

***

Mentally, almost any activity can provide the same meditative and mind calming affects, if done with "Mindfulness.

***

Spiritually, any form of prayer can produce all of the same benefits. Jesus said: Ask and you shall receive. (Matthew 7:7-8).

***

So why practice Tai Chi? First of all, it combines all of the above benefits into one activity. Secondly, it can be enjoyed by almost anyone, at any time, and at any place. Lastly, it's a beautiful Art that provides an immense opportunity for self- expression, personal growth, and a venue for infinite research of an age-old tradition.

***

TAI CHI CLASSICS

Without knowledge of the Classics, you will only be performing a Tai Chi like exercise and not true Tai Chi (Cheng 1991).

***

If one who is learning Tai Chi does not practice according to the principles of the Classics, they will not experience the essential significance and effects of Tai Chi (Soong 1995).

***

The Tai chi Classics are a collection of over 100 articles, written by Master practitioners over the centuries. They cover everything from philosophical principles, to methods of practice and application. Previously passed down in secret from generation to generation, they became public starting in the mid-1930s. They have been authenticated and have served as one of the most important guides for the study of Tai Chi. This document is based on the thoughts and theories as they have been interpreted from the Tai Chi Classics.

***

Following are several sources known to be Tai Chi Classics.
TAI CHI TREATISE by Hui Shih (ca. 300 BC).
THEORY ON TAI CHI CHUAN by Wang Tsung-Yueh (ca. 1800 AD).
TREATISE by Master Yang Chen-Fu (ca. 1800 AD).
SONG OF THE THIRTEEN POSTURES by Unknow author (n.d.).
EXPOSITION OF INSIGHT INTO THE PRACTICE OF THE THIRTEEN POSTURES by Wu Yu-Hsiang (ca. 1800 AD).
TREATISE by Master Wong Chung-Yua (ca. 1600 AD).
TREATISE ON THE PRACTICE OF THE THIRTEEN POSTURES by Master Wu Yu-Hsiang (ca. 1850 AD).
THE EIGHT TRUTHS OF TAI CHI by Unknow author (n.d.).

TAI CHI CHUAN CHING by Grand Master Chang San-Feng (ca. 1200 AD).

TREATISE ON TAI CHI CHUAN by Wang Tsung Yueh (ca. 1800AD).

YANG'S TEN IMPORTANT POINTS by Yang Cheng-fu (ca. 1850 AD).

SONG OF THE EIGHT POSTURES attributed to T'an Meng-hsien (n.d.).

FIVE CHARACTER SECRET by Li I-Yu (ca. 1900 AD).

***

Several of the Classics are very brief and quite obscure because they were written as prompts to help students remember what they were taught orally by their teacher. Therefore, in many occasions it may be necessary to dig a lot deeper and find commentaries to get the true intent of what was written. It is best to try and use resources that have a direct linkage to the original author. There are plenty of books and web sites to meet this need.

INTERPRETATION

Trying to explain the philosophy of Tai Chi is inevitably confounded by words. Through practice and study, we must experience the truth for ourselves, as a way to comprehend the words and explanations of others.

***

A lot of the original Tai Chi documents were written in a poetic style. They required an oral interpretation by a competent instructor to be understood.

***

Traditional Chinese writing was not punctuated, and it was the reader's job to parse the sentence. How a person perceives which clauses are subordinate and how to match subjects and predicates, can determine the meaning of a passage. Therefore, when reading traditional or contemporary material related to Tai Chi, certain techniques and theories will only make sense if you rearrange the existing sentence structure.

***

In order to study Tai Chi, you must find correct explanations. (Wang 15th Century AD).

***

Many of the concepts, techniques, and teachings of Tai Chi can be confusing, contradictory and misleading when taken literally. There are several reasons for this problem. First and foremost is the issue of Translation. Chinese characters often have various meanings for the same character and can easily be misinterpreted. Often, the person who is translating an oral interview from Chinese to English will make a minor mistake that can alter the original context. Furthermore, many of the Traditional Chinese teachers did not want to share their knowledge with non-family members and especially foreigners. Therefore, they only revealed a few fundamentals and hid the meaning of some of the more important elements. Also, written errors in the Tai Chi Classic were sometimes intentional in order to hide the true meaning. Lastly, many authors who attempt to interpret and translate original text are influenced by their personal bias and perimeters. In conclusion, anyone who wishes to study and practice the art of Tai Chi must approach it as a scholar. Thus, you will be able to filter out the true meaning of the techniques and tailor a practice that reflects your personal style.

***

Teachings that are based on universal truths, will be easy to understand and easier to put into practice (Lao Tzu 5th Century AD).

***

The teachings and techniques of Tai Chi are filled with paradox and contradictions. Some contemporary authors use paraphrasing to help remove direct contradictions, but occasionally this result in the original intent being altered.

***

PURPOSE OF TAI CHI

The most significant benefit is to transfer the meditative tranquility achieved by practicing Tai Chi into how we respond to others on a daily basis. The Tai Chi Classics state: To develop one's spiritual being is the real contribution of Tai Chi (Yang B.H. 19th Century AD).

***

The ultimate purpose of Tai Chi is to provide us with wisdom and insights that we can apply to life. If we can't do that, then it doesn't matter how well we perform the movements and postures. True Tai Chi must be lived (Lin 1964).

***

The Theory is to help people attain longevity and rejuvenation. The techniques and form are the least things to be concerned with (Yang L.-C. 18th Century AD).

***

The intention of Tai Chi is to rejuvenate the body, prolong good health, and encourage us to act with compassion towards all things.

***

The physical benefits are similar to other forms of exercise, especially yoga. Along with improving muscle tone, this gentle exercise effects the circulatory, respiratory, and nervous system.

***

To have health in our senior years has become a major priority as modern medicine has extended the average life expectancy. In order to enjoy these additional years, one has to be healthy and capable of recuperating from medical procedures. Perhaps one of the most significant benefits of Tai Chi is express in the ancient adage "Long life, but not old". A more contemporary expression would be "Youthfulness within old age".

FORM / FUNCTION

FORM is practicing the sequence of Tai chi movements as an exercise by uniting the various postures into one continuous flow.

***

FUNCTION is adapting the FORM into maneuvers that can be applied as self-defense techniques. Push Hands, Applications, and Sparring are examples of FUNCTION.

***

Tai Chi was created to prevent illness and promote longevity. The Form is essential while the martial Functions are secondary (Song of The Thirteen Postures (n.d.).

***

In Tai Chi there is Form, also called Structure, Essence, or Theory. Likewise, there is Function, Practical Use, and Application.

***

Tai Chi Chuan is the correct term to describe the art that is being addressed in this document. Tai Chi Chuan literally means "Grand Ultimate Fist". In Western vernacular, it would be translated as "The Fist of God". Tai Chi Chuan can be practice as a martial art. It is specifically referred to as an Internal, soft style of Kung Fu.

***

However, the purpose of this booklet is to omit the martial arts applications, and only offer thoughts and theories that will help the reader defend themselves against unnecessary accidents, poor health and premature aging. Therefore, the term Tai Chi Chuan will be modified to Tai Ch for the duration of this essay to stress the emphasis on FORM rather than FUNCTION.

THE SPIRITUAL PHILOSOPHY OF SHEN

The Chinese character for Shen has a variety of meanings such as: spirit, soul, mind, God, and Deity. Like Yin and Yang, they change depending on the context of the material.

***

Shen is that aspect of our being that we refer to as Spiritual. It embodies consciousness and thought. It is through Shen that we radiate ourselves to the world. Shen draws our attention to the Divine. Shen can be strengthened thru the practice of Tai Chi.

***

Shen is spiritual consciousness. It is an awareness of the Power that permeates the Universe. It is innate at birth but often lost to one's Ego or ordinary consciousness (Wen 1973). It can be rediscovered through many ways, including the Tai Chi.

***

Tai Chi is different from most other forms of exercise because of its Spiritual component which emphasizes doing the right thing in your daily activities. Mechanics related to the practice are secondary. The primary activity is to use the mind to acknowledge the Divine's presence within our body. One of the techniques for doing this is to imagine swallowing in Heaven's energy and channel it to the Tan Tien (Cheng 1999).

***

The five major styles of Tai Chi: CHEN, YANG, WU, WOO, and SUN are similar at their core. The movements, sequence, and names of the postures vary among the various styles, but all are founded on the same basic Spiritual principles. First, acknowledge God in all things. Vast indeed is the scope of the greatness of the Creative Basis. All things and all beings originate from it (I CHING: #1). Secondly, Live Life as a testament to Scripture. All day long I'll praise and honor you, O God, for all that you have done for me (Psalms 71:8).

***

The desire is to help people attain longevity and Spiritual rejuvenation. The techniques and Forms of Tai Chi are the least things to be concerned with. (Song of The Thirteen Postures (n.d.).

***

The mind should depend on the Spirit, not the Chi (Cheng 1985).

***

Tai Chi pays tribute to the cosmological framework it is based on. It is a symbolic prayer that is accomplished through movement. The first posture pays homage to Heaven and the last posture is representational of an "A Men" at the end of a prayer (Yang 20th Century AD).

***

Tai Chi can become a blessing to Man when this exercise is integrated with a high moral purpose and spiritual value (Wen 1973).

***

Yang Ban Hou emphasizes the greatest application of Chi for the whole body is to raise spiritual consciousness. (Yang, C.-Fu 20th Century AD).

***

Arouse the Spirit and there is no reason for anxiety about clumsiness (Wu 19th Century).

***

In the practice of Tai Chi, the main thing is the Spirit. (Yang C.-F. 20th Century AD).

***

Chi fills the body with its presence while the spirit controls it.

***

By applying the concepts of Heaven in seeking the goals of Tai Chi, everything will eventually come about and happen naturally (Tung 20th Century).

***

Relax. Give up. Yield. One must yield to the Divine. Relax and merge into unity with the Infinite. This is described as the integration of Heaven, Earth, and Man (Yang C.-F. 20th Century AD).

***

Be Rooted in the Oneness of the Tao. (Lao Tzu 5th Century AD).

***

The Wind and I are One. Wed your breath with ours and know the meaning of Life.

***

True Tai Chi is letting go of appearances while practicing the Form. Perform each movement naturally and allow your being to merge with the Divine.

***

As one's practice advances, attention to the details of the form can be dispensed with because the spiritual aspects of Tai Chi presuppose the practical. One must ascent from the practical craft of performing the postures to the artistic, philosophical, and spiritual possibilities (Soong 1995).

***

Practicing the form without knowledge of the Spiritual concepts that are the foundation of Tai Chi, is similar to using Regular gas to run your vehicle. When you add the Spiritual aspects, you are switching to Highest. Un-caffeinated to Caffeinated.

***

Tai chi is the way of Life and the way of Life is Love. Love all things equally, Heaven and Earth are one body (Hui 3rd Century BC).

***

Tai Chi evolved from the "Ultimateless", the origin of movement and quietude, and the Mother of all things (Wang 15th Century)

***

Inwardly make the Shen (Spirit) strong and outwardly exhibit calmness and peace (Wu 19th Century AD).

***

If Essence and Spirit can be raised, then there is no need for concern with being slow and awkward (Wu 19th Century AD).

***

Do not be concerned with Form. It's best to forget your own existence (The Eight Truths of Tai Chi (n.d.).

***

Your own soul is nourished when you are kind to others. (Proverbs 11:17)

***

Humility is an expression of Spiritual maturity.

***

The I-CHING (9th Century AD) states that great success comes through for the honest and true.

***

Accomplish much without doing. Act by not acting is called Non-Action or Wu- Wei. Become an empty vehicle for the Divine to act through you (Lao Tzu 5th Century AD).

***

Restrain your Ego while practicing. Thus, the Ego is not responsible for the action but instead imagine it is Divine intervention that accomplishes what is needed to be done.

***

The philosophy of Oneness allows the Ego to expand beyond its' self and experience a connection to all things.

***

Enlightenment is something already inside all Beings. It is the deluded mind that presents one from awakening (Buddha (tr.) 1993).

***

Tai Chi has its roots in the I-Ching. The *TEN WINGS* (a commentary on the I-CHING by Confucius) describes the I-Ching as a symbolic document rich in moral and spiritual content. The *GREAT COMMENTARY* states that the I-Ching offers a spiritual experience that allows the individual to understand the deeper patterns of the Universe.

***

A central doctrine of Tai Chi is to physically and mentally be in harmony with the Universe.

***

Tai Chi is activity through spiritual meditation.

***

The Tai Chi Classics are founded on three major principles. First, it should be performed as a symbolic prayer that acknowledges the Divine created all things and is always present in them. Secondly, live your life in a moral and correct way. Lastly, practice and study will lead to a longer and healthier life (Waysun 1990).

***

The entire world is but one vital energy. Use the concept of Chi to realize the fundamental oneness of all existence and stop seeing yourself as separate (Chuang-Tzu 4th Century BC).

***

Yin comes from Heaven and Yang comes from Earth. When both intermingle and join, all things come forth (Chuang-Tzu, 4th Century BC).

***

Though imagination and knowledge, learn to expand your boundaries to include the cosmic process (Chuang-Tzu, 4th Century BC).

***

The more we physically embody the spiritual doctrines of Tai Chi while practicing, the more we can adapt them to our daily lives (Chuang-Tzu 4th Century BC).

***

The ancient Chinese medical text *HUANGDI-NEIJING-LINGSHU* states that Heaven abides so that we have virtue. Earth abides so that we have Chi. When virtue flows and Chi is blended, there is Shen (Chuang 4th Century BC). This is one of the most significant reoccurring spiritual doctrines of Tai Chi. It involves the creation of Shen by combining innate physical Chi with external spiritual beliefs.

***

How does Tai Chi create Shen? A simplified explanation of how to accomplish this is as following: Root the body from the waist down, to absorb the energy from the Earth (Yang/positive) and empty the body from the waist up, so the energy from Heaven may enter (Yin/negative). Both energies meet in the center at the waist level in the Tan Tien. The heat generated from the activity of the legs combines the two and produces Shen, an enhanced form of Chi.

***

By adhering to the Spiritual philosophy of Tai Chi, one's enhanced Chi is transformed into Shen. The energy generated by Shen will automatically be used to help maintain and rejuvenate the physical body. However, more important is to direct the

Mind to manifest Shen as a tangible compassion for all things. "I shall not kill" (Exodus 20:13). "Kill no living thing" (Buddha (ed.)1993). "The Lord is gracious and righteous; our God is full of compassion" (Psalm 116:5). "Heavens way is to benefit and do no harm" (Lao Tzu 4th Century AD). The next time you find a harmless insect in your house, let it live. It only takes a little extra time to remove it safely. How does it make you feel to be in control of a life/death decision over one of God's creatures?

***

Master Da Liu in his book *TAI CHI CHUAN & MEDITATION* (1991) states Tai Chi can be experienced as an Alchemical procedure that enhances Spiritual awareness. It refines one psychic substance into another. It's a belief system that involves the act of inhaling air which you believe is permeated with GOD'S essence and combing it with your Bioelectrical/Chi in the Tan Tien/Center, to generate a spiritual product called Shen.

***

Tai Chi, as well as being an exercise in control, concentration, and grace, also has deep spiritual meaning. Many of the movements are symbolic of refurbishing the soul and attaining inner peace. This is expressed in more detail in The Eight Trigrams of Tai Chi.

***

The Tai Chi Classics state that Shen should help propel the body during Tai Chi and not muscular force. It will also contribute to good health. If you approach this exercise as a form of Prayer, you will enhance the many benefits that result from frequent practice.

***

The *TAO TE CHING* by Lao Tzu is one of the most important interpretations of the I-CHING ever translated. The Tai Chi Classics consistently refer to the principles established in this document. The emphasis is on acknowledging God (The Way) as the Creator of all things, replacing our Ego with God's essence while performing Tai Chi, and applying the teachings from the *TAO TE CHING* to how we interact with others.

***

Practicing and studying Tai Chi for only a few minutes a day will motivate you to transfer the concepts to other daily activities that will have a cumulative impact on improving your health. For example, along with focusing on good posture while performing the movements, you can make an effort to continuing practicing good posture as you go through your daily activities. This applies to breathing, balance, mindfulness, walking, diet, and most important, an awareness of God's presence.

***

THE NECESSITY OF FAITH

Tai Chi does not attempt to convert or convince the practitioner to any set of religious doctrines. Tai Chi does not proselytize, instead it reinforces philosophically the fundamental themes that permeate all major world religions. The notion that the Divine is in everything and all of Creation is somehow interconnected are universal ideas. Furthermore, human logic alone is not a sufficient tool for comprehending Divine truths, it requires Faith. Adopting an open mind toward the practices of others does not represent a betrayal of one's beliefs. Instead, it is a reminder that we are all in the same boat; we are born, we live, and we die.

***

Faith can be described as complete trust or confidence in something that is not based on proof. Even though it is unseen, the believer has a conviction that what they expect will come to pass.

***

If you have a host of hens but lack a rooster, how will you get eggs? Similarly, you can be well educated in the practice of Tai Chi but without Faith, it will be fruitless (Chuang 3rd Century BC).

***

Tai Chi is externally Invisible but Internally Rejuvenating.

***

It is a process that produces results but is not fully understood. Consequently, certain aspects are apt to be labeled Metaphysical (Wen 1973).

***

The principles exist and the benefits will follow (Cheng 1981).

This truth is confirmed by the many who regularly practice Tai Chi.

***

One must yield to the Divine. Relax and merge into unity with the Infinite. This is described as the integration of Heaven and Earth (Yang C.-F. 2005).

***

The Tai Chi principle is as simple as this: yield yourself to the power of the Universe. Tai Chi is born out of Infinity (Wong 16th Century AD).

***

So indistinct it seems not to exist. The indistinct nature of Tai Chi refers to the fact that we may not perceive results directly but will still benefit from its essence if we have faith in its' principles. Just as we cannot see gravity itself but only the effects of falling objects (Lin 1964).

***

After a few weeks of external exercise (aerobics, weight lifting, calisthenics, etc.) you'll usually notice external changes, such as weight loss, increased endurance and improved muscle tone. However, after a few weeks of practicing Tai Chi the results are much less visible because it is designed to improve those aspects of your body that are internal and can't be seen. People don't die because of a lack of muscle tone or a few extra pounds. They die from organ failure, blocked arteries, and other internal complications. These are conditions that Tai Chi has a reputation for impacting. Do not get discouraged If you don't see any apparent external visible improvements. Have Faith and just keep at it!

***

Success will come through for the honest and true (I-Ching (tr.) 2017).

***

While performing Tai Chi, have faith that God will help generate the benefits associated with this exercise as you integrate the spiritual and philosophical aspects into your practice and daily life. Five to fifteen minutes of practice, four or five times a week will provide many benefits. Do not get attached to seeing external changes or feeling internal Bioelectricity /Chi.

***

Mastery of Tai Chi is achieved by letting things take their own course (Lao Tzu 5th Century AD). Go with the flow.

***

Wu-Wei is a powerful principle based on Faith. While practicing Tai Chi, the idea is to focus on the process and not the results. Practice diligently without being attached to specific results or benefits.

***

Wu-Wei is having Faith that the expected outcomes will occur without the Ego striving to make it happen.

***

PERSONAL STYLE

The more you read and study the art of Tai Chi, the more you will be able to tailor the vast amount of information and techniques into your personal style.

***

Do not seek to follow in the footsteps of the men of old; seek what they sought (Basho 16thCentury AD). No need to emulate a Master's style, instead seek knowledge in the Tai Chi Classics and *Tao Te Ching* as they did.

***

It is not necessary to imitate any particular FORM or Instructor verbatim. Instead, focus on developing your own style based on what you feel instead of what you look like.

***

It's important to listen and respond to what your body and innate feelings suggest.

***

After comprehending the fundamentals, the more you practice, the grater will be your own ingenious refinements (Wang 15th Century AD).

***

Although there are innumerable variations, the principles that pervade them remain the same (Wang 15th Century AD).

***

No two people seem to be doing the exact same form. This is to be expected, as no two person's energy is the same. The small artistic

differences are inconsequential, as long as the concepts are correct (Tchoung 21st Century).

***

Listen to your body and let your body tell you what is right (Wang
15th Century AD).

***

Tai Chi is an internal exercise. Do not be attached to what your
practice looks like externally.

***

Transcend the limitations of techniques. Put aside all notions of
displaying skill or proper appearance.

***

Due to the difference in body type and predisposition, everyone
will impart their own essence to the art of Tai Chi. The small artistic differences are inconsequential. As long as the concepts are
correct, the benefits will follow (Yang Z.-D. 21st Century AD).

***

Escape from the bonds of a particular style and experience the joy
and benefits of just practicing (Lee 1975).

***

Be aware of how your body feels. Don't strain or force any of the
mechanics or techniques. Instead, accept your physical limitations. Your "Mindfulness", "Philosophy", and "Right Living" will
compensate for any physical restraints.

***

Eliminate comparisons.

***

Great skill may look clumsy and the greatest perfection can look
imperfect (I-Ching (tr.) 2017).

***

The important benefits are not obtained in the detail appearance of the Form, but must be sought in the principles that the Form expresses (Cheng 1994).

***

Do not be concerned about what you look like externally while practicing. Some of your movements will be performed well and some won't. Accepting the imperfections of your practice will make your Tai Chi "whole/complete". YIN is imperfection and YANG is perfection. Together they form a "whole/complete" experience.

***

PHYSICAL / METAPHYSICAL

Tai Chi is composed equally of Physical and Metaphysical concepts. Both are needed to implement the various techniques involved in the study and practice of this intriguing art. Following are simplified definitions of each, as they relate to Tai Chi.

***

When something is Physical, it is really there. It has a material existence that is perceptible through the senses and subject to the Laws of Nature. Tai Chi would describe this Physical reality as being Yang or having the characteristics of being substantial, solid, palpable, observable, and of the Earth.

***

Many of the physical benefits of Tai Chi correspond directly to specific Physical techniques. A few examples: Shifting most of your weight on to one leg will improve your balance and strengthen your lower body. Keeping your spine erect during practice should aid with maintaining good posture and blood circulation. The various movements of the arms and legs tend to lubricate joints and loosen muscles. In general, daily practice results in an overall feeling of wellbeing. These are all Physical conditions that are tangible through the senses and could be quantified with appropriate testing.

***

In the opposite realm are Metaphysical concepts. They involve the relationships between Mind and Matter. It is the philosophy of what is possible outside of objective reality. It includes experiences beyond the observable physical universe. It is that aspect of existence that cannot be observed or measured. Tai Chi refers to the Metaphysical as being Yin and having the traits of being insubstantial, ethereal, subjective, theoretical, and of Heaven.

***

In Tai Chi the Metaphysical theories surround several major ideas. The first and foremost is Faith. Tai Chi is founded on the concept that there is a Divine Cosmic energy that pervades all Matter and Non-Matter, which unites all things through the philosophy of Oneness. Furthermore, this Divine Cosmic energy can be acknowledged within the human body and used in multiple ways. This includes concepts that combine the Mind with Faith to initiate techniques that will expand and influence our energy. Another major Metaphysical theory is the existence of the Tan Tien or Psychic Center in the lower abdomen. This is an imaginary caldron where the Mind brings together specific Body energies to produce an elixir that is responsible for benefits particular to Tai Chi.

***

A fundamental fact proclaimed by practitioners of Tai Chi is; Physical components must be proportionately integrated with Metaphysical aspects in order to receive Tai Chi's many unique benefits.

***

This is only a brief introduction to the interwoven characteristics of the Physical and Metaphysical theories of Tai Chi. With study, the practitioner will come to comprehend the application of these two very important principles that blend Body and Mind. The beauty of Tai Chi occurs when these two opposite realities are successfully combined into one.

***

A word of caution. Don't be misled by instructors who promise supernatural results if you study their particular school of Tai Chi. They often require years of instruction, esoteric techniques, and payment. There are people who are born with innate gifts and have cultivated them. This has enables them to do extraordinary feats using their Chi. However, most of these individuals will acknowledge it is a gift and not something that can be taught. Beware of Charlatans!

***

TAI CHI & SCIENCE

One of Tai Chi's most unique benefits is its' positive effect on our internal organs/systems as a result of increasing our Bioelectricity/Chi and its' flow. This is not something you can see or measure, without the aid of equipment such as a Voltmeter or PH Meter. However, many cardio exercise machines do measure the wattage output you generate while exercising. If you understand the physical mechanics of how this process occurs, you can be confident that you are generating Bioelectricity/Chi when you practice Tai Chi. Again, being aware that something is happening even though you can't see it is extremely important towards making a commitment to continue practicing Tai Chi.

***

The human body at rest generates approximately 100 watts a day. An athlete can produce more than 1000 watts a day. This Bioelectricity/Chi makes the heart beat, the brain function, muscles contract, helps creates new cells, and much more.

***

Dr. Jerry Tennat developed a Biomodulator Device (TENS) that is an electrical stimulator that supplements the human body with additional electricity to treat various physiological health problems. In his book *HEALING IS VOLTAGE* he makes the following statements: Your body runs on electricity. To maintain good health, you need the appropriate voltage (-50mV) to help generate new cell growth (Tennat 2010).

***

In 2015 the Samueli Institute for Information Biology did a clinical trial and one of the findings stated that your body naturally generates electricity via muscle activity and breathing. Dr. Ernest Gardner in his book *FUNDAMENTALS OF NEUROLOGY* (1959) presented this concept: Using visualization to send an idea about generating electricity to a certain spot, will affect the electrons in that region.

***

Following are scientific facts based on current research:

1. <u>Muscle activity</u>. When you engage your muscles, electrons are emitted. This is called "Piezoelectricity".

2. <u>Breathing</u>. Oxygen is one of the requirements needed to Charge the electrons of the body.

3. <u>Visualization.</u> Influences the Charge of electrons and electrical flow within the human body.

***

A fundamental concept of Tai Chi is that a practitioner can improve/maintain their health via increasing the level and flow of their Bioelectricity/Chi. This is done by incorporating the following Tai Chi principles, which correspond to the above scientific facts:

1. <u>Muscle activity:</u> Shifting the body weight from one thigh muscle to the other, generates electrons or "Piezoelectricity".

2. <u>Breathing:</u> Increasing oxygen via breathing enhances the Charge to the electrons of the body.

3. <u>Visualization:</u> Imagining that one's innate Bioelectricity/Chi mixed with breathing along with an awareness of the Divine, increases the Charge and flow of electrons. Enhanced Bioelectricity/Chi is known as Shen in Tai Chi.

***

CHI

Chi is one of the more evasive concepts associated with Tai Chi. There are a great variety of explanations and definitions. There are at least 30 different meanings for the Chinese character Chi. A few examples are "air", "gas", "breath", "spirit", "vigor", "energy", "nourishment", "life force", etc. Furthermore, the original intent of the word has evolved over the last 3000 years. The best suggestion is to research the term and construct your own definition. However, remain flexible and tolerant towards those who have beliefs about Chi that differ from yours. Furthermore, it's best to forget about Chi while practicing the form and adapt the philosophy that Chi will do its work without conscious effort of the Ego.

***

Don't be misled by the various suggestions on how to increase, feel and manipulate the Chi in your body. There are many intricate techniques professed by modern day teachers who claim that their methods will lead to getting in contact with your Chi. The simple truth is you don't have to feel or experience anything. You just have to adhere to the philosophy that if you combine frequent practice with "Right Living" and Faith, your Chi will be enhanced and you will receive the benefits associated with Tai Chi.

***

There are various aspects of Chi. Spirit and Essence are two of the most prominent. Spirit is a subtler level of vital energy. Essence is its thicker, more tangible form. An example of Spirit Chi would be the vapors that permeate the body or the electricity that flows through the Meridians. It is often referred to as Shen. Essence Chi or internal Innate Chi is associated with blood and other bodily fluids (Chuang 4th Century BC).

***

Chi is an invisible force known only by its effects. Health and longevity are two of the greatest side effects of its unobstructed flow.

***

Chi pervades and connects everything.

***

It can be augmented by careful exercise and "Right Living".

***

Chi is a vital force, a type of electricity.

***

Piezoelectricity in the human body is the electrical charge that is generated by muscular movement. When you engage your muscles, electrons are emitted.

***

Chi is an innate bioelectricity that can be influence by the Mind, exercise, diet, and "Right Living".

***

The Tai Chi Classics state to use the Mind via imagination to gather the Chi in the Tan Tien. Then without conscious effort, allow Shen Chi to move the body, instead of muscular force.

***

Gravity, the Magnetic pull of the North Pole, and static electricity in the air, are all factors that impact the external Chi found in nature.

***

Feeling Chi is temporary. Yet, know the unknown is knowable, then move on (Shaw, 2002).

***

The Chi in the body may sometimes appear and sometimes disappear (Wang 15th Century AD).

***

Chi exist in the body without being explicitly noticed (Soong 1995)).

***

The contradictory expression "No Chi" is a common metaphor in Tai Chi. It does not refer to the absence of Chi, but rather a conscious effort to let Chi work on its own, without any guidance or expectations. The theory of "No Chi" allows one's Spirit to determine when and how it is use (Cheng 1994). To clarify this concept, Shen Chi (also called Spirit) is the product of combining one's internal Innate Chi with external Natural Chi in the Tan Tien. Without conscious effort, portions of Shen Chi will be used to propel movements, address existing medical issues, or be stored in the body for future use. Also, it can give us the moral strength to deal with Life in a more compassionate manner.

***

Chi already exists in each cell. Chi is present in all things at all times. Acknowledge its' existence and potential.

***

Don't be concerned about feeling your Chi. Instead, accept the fact that it is present. It's your awareness of its' existence that will have an impact.

***

One's personal internal Chi is vitalized by the integration of the external Chi that is all around us.

***

External Natural Chi can be influenced by one's Karma. Humility and "Right Living" generates positive Chi.

***

Think often of the Chi collecting in the Tan Tien. The Tan Tien is like a stove and the twisting of the waist is like a bellows. Here the

Chi will be stoked and heated. The heated Chi will permeate the body like steam or perspiration without conscious intent.

***

There are three types of Chi. First is Innate Chi. This is the Chi that you are born with and is always with you. The second is Nature Chi. This is the Chi that exist in all things outside of the body. The third is Shen Chi. It is made by combining Innate Chi and Nature Chi in the Tan Tien. This is the Chi that is used to mobilize movement during practice, aid in rejuvenation of one's health, and stored in the body for future benefits (Cheng 1981).

***

Chi is like a vapor. Barley seen but always present. Use it wisely (Lao Tzu 5th Century AD).

***

Chi is the electrometric energy found in all Matter.

***

The Tai Chi Classics emphasize that acknowledging the Divine within us is more important than experiencing the presents of Chi. Our bodies will automatically use our Chi where and when it is required.

***

Be content to feel Chi at intervals. Now you feel it and now you don't. Yin/Yang.

***

How can you be totally relaxed while practicing if you are preoccupied with focusing on feeling your Chi? Instead, focus on the fundamentals and Chi will take care of its self. This is a primary doctrine of Tai Chi.

***

Keep the Tail Bone straight so the Chi can raise from the center (Tan Tien) and go up the spine towards the crown of the head. The flow will continue to the hands, if the shoulders, elbows, and wrist are unlocked and relaxed.

***

Chinese medicine thinks of muscles as containing Chi. When the muscle is relaxed the Chi can be dispersed. Chi is present in all living things (Chang 12th Century AD).

***

Intercourse between Heaven and Earth creates Man. The two intertwine forming a harmony and as a result, things are born (Dong 1st Century BC). There are various interpretations of how Chi can be augmented based on this original symbolic explanation. Following is one way to transfer this esoteric elixir into a practical physical application. A basic concept in Tai Chi states the following: From the waist up the body is symbolic of Heaven (Insubstantial-empty-relaxed-negative-Yin). The spine is straight, shoulders relaxed, elbow and wrist joints are unlocked. From the waist down the body is symbolic of Earth (Substantial-full-heavy-tense-positive-Yang). The feet are rooted, knees are bent, and the leg muscles are tense. Next, think in terms of creating electricity by mixing negative electrons (generated by upper body mechanics) with positive electrons (generated by lower body mechanics). When "opposites" meet in the center (Tan Tien), something happens; heat is generated. Furthermore, with proper thoughts and techniques, Chi can be transformed to Shen.

***

The upper body is soft and relaxed (Yin), while the lower body is firm and rooted (Yang). When opposites come together in the center, there is an event. Heat is generated and the Chi is aroused (Soong 1995).

***

In sitting or reclined Meditation that are practiced in stillness, a popular technique is to use the mind to circulate the Chi or channel it to a specific area. However, during Tai Chi movements do not use the Ego to direct the Chi. This creates stress related to expectations. The Chi will move on its own if you implement the proper techniques during practice.

***

Though out the whole body the intent should be on the Spirit and not the Chi. If it is on the Chi there will be stagnation. One who has it on the Chi will have no strength but one who does not have it on the Chi will be strong (Wu 19th Century AD). This statement presents a paradox to what many others say regarding the use of Chi. So, what is the true meaning of this oxymoron? Master Yang Cheng Fu explains that instead of consciously using Chi, follow the principle of Wu-Wei (Non-Action). This notion of not using Chi is an example of allowing the Spirit to act; and decide how best to use your Chi.

***

SUBSTANTIAL / INSUBSTANTIAL

While practicing Tai Chi, things fluctuate between Substantial (Yang/positive) and Insubstantial (Yin/negative). Change is constant. Substantial and Insubstantial must be clearly distinguished (Yang C.-F. 20th Century).

***

Corresponding with Yin/Yang are Substantial/Insubstantial. From the waist up the body is Insubstantial and from the waist down it is Substantial. This is a priority and should be understood and maintained. Also, there are subdivisions within each element. Extremely important is the subdivision of Yang/Substantial below the waist. The leg that supports most of the body weight is the Substantial leg and the leg that has very little or no weight is the Insubstantial leg. The constant shifting of the legs from Substantial to Insubstantial is what generates the heat that fuels the Tan Tien. Not as important, is the subdivision above the waist. One arm is classified as Substantial and the other is Insubstantial. However, both arms should remain relaxed, loose, light, and empty of any tension. The differentiation involving the arms is only significant in the application of Function and Push Hands.

***

The Substantial leg should be as heavy as a mountain (Wang 18th Century AD)

***

Gravity extends to the center of the earth. Gravity automatically roots your foot in the Substantial leg. Use your imagination to get the feeling of being rooted to the earth.

***

Focus on being balanced and stable on the Substantial leg at the end of each posture. When necessary, use the Insubstantial leg to assist.

***

Shift the weight back and forth from Substantial to Insubstantial (full to empty-positive to negative- Yin to Yang). This will generate energy. This energy from the Earth will find its way to the Tan Tien, and be transformed to heat.

***

BREATHING

The Ancient Sages understood the intimate connection between the flow of breath and the currents of energy that animate the body and raise consciousness. They learned to utilize the breath both naturally and deliberately. They considered it to be one of the most relevant components of Tai Chi.

***

Practice without conscious control of the Breath. Conscious control can lead to clumsiness of movement. Breath naturally. This allows the mind to focus on other aspects of Tai Chi (Soong 1995).

***

Being able to breath naturally leads to agility (Wu 19th Century AD).

***

One must breath naturally; then the mind will be alert and movements will be natural. If one pays conscious attention to the breathing, the movements will be dull and ineffective (Wang 18th Century AD).

***

Free and unrestrained breathing is best.

***

Coercing the breath is unnatural (Lao Tzu 5th Century AD).

***

Some modern-day instructors teach numerous theories on the best way to breath while practicing Tai Chi. Many promote their personal techniques of breathing that they claim will enhance the various benefits and aspects associated with Tai Chi. Some of their suggestions are appropriate for other forms of meditations or exercise but should not be applied to Tai Chi. A very common technique that they promote, is to inhale as you begin the movement and exhale as you finish the movement. This is not a good idea because it forces you to define the timing of the movement based on your breathing pattern, instead of letting the movement determine the flow of breath. Furthermore, some movements vary in length and time duration. For example, the movement "raise hands" can be performed by inhaling one breath as you raise your hands up and exhale one breath as you lower your hands. However, a more involved movement such as "Single Whip" may take several inhalations and exhalations to correctly complete the form. Furthermore, if you adhere to the theory to move as slow as possible, this can require multiple breaths for the most basic movements, such as Homage to Heaven. Therefore, stick to what the Classics have recommending for 3000 years. There is no need to coordinate breathing with movement. Instead, just focus on performing the movements and forget about attempting to establish a controlled breathing pattern. Just breath naturally.

***

Trying to coordinate breathing with movement will interrupt your attempt at relaxing the mind and body.

***

Once the form has been memorized and muscle memory reduces the need to concentrate on what comes next in the sequence, you may become aware that you are subconsciously coordinating certain movements with corresponding breathing patterns that occur naturally. You will find that specific movements encourage an inhalation and other movements naturally allow for an exhalation. This is not the same as consciously forcing an inhalation or an exhalation to coincide with a particular movement. You may also notice that the time it takes to inhale or exhale may vary greatly, depending on the movement. Furthermore, it's ok to use small quick breaths to adjust your breathing so it can flow naturally with the movement.

***

The important concept is to breath naturally and not allow your breathing pattern to distract you from performing Tai Chi with "Mindfulness".

***

If your movements are relaxed and your breathing is relaxed, they will unite as "one" because they are sharing the same concept of "Relaxation".

***

Don't try to control breathing. Just relax and breath according to the natural flow of the movement.

***

The most important principle related to Tai Chi breathing is to maintain a relaxed pattern of breathing, Tai Chi is based on concepts and principles that are designed to eliminate stress while performing the exercise. Forced breathing will cause stress.

***

POSTURES

Ninety percent of the postures require the following body alignment:

1. Neck and spine straight.
2. Knees and elbows slightly bent.
3. Slightly tuck your tail bone. This will help make you aware of your Tan Tien or Center.
4. Having most of the body weight on one leg only.

***

A fundamental concept of Tai Chi is to imagine being hung from Heaven by the top of your head with invisible thread. This concept allows you to experience body lightness, freedom of movement, and improved balance. Furthermore, it symbolically establishes a bond between the individual and Heaven/God.

***

Regardless of the recommended body alignment for a Posture, adjust your feet and body accordingly. This will help maintain a feeling of comfort and balance. You don't break the flow when you pause to adjust your body, you break the flow when you let your mind wander outside of Tai Chi principles. Maintaining control of your thoughts is an important concept In Tai Chi.

***

Postures performed according to your individual style are considered correct if they are comfortable. Reduce stress by not straining. Therefore, the suggestions for foot and hand placements are to be interpreted as approximations and not strict rules. The Golden Rule is to make adjustments based on what feels comfortable.

***

All Postures involve arm and hand placement. There are too many variations to describe in this manual. However, there is one fundamental principle that applies to almost every arm and hand position. Relax and unlock shoulder, elbow, and wrist joints. Both arms and hands should feel empty, light, loose, ethereal; similar to a Rag Doll. Relaxing the upper torso and limbs is what allows the Chi to flow from the Tan Tien to the finger tips.

***

All Posture are rooted in the feet and legs. At the end of each movement you will be in either a Front or Back stance. Occasionally you will assume a Transitional stance that occurs between postures. Regardless of your stance, it should be comfortable and allow you to move easily in any direction.

***

The 3 basic body Stances only describe where your legs and feet should be positioned when you arrive at a posture. There is a variety of movements that get you from one stance to the next. Don't think of the postures as being static, even though you can pause briefly at the end to feel for stability, balanced, and alignment.

1. <u>Front Stance</u>. The front foot is pointed straight ahead and bears approximately 70-95 % of the body weight. This makes the front leg Full or Substantial. The back foot is at a 45-degree angle to the front foot and bears about 5-30% of the body weight. This makes the back leg Empty or Insubstantial. The feet are about shoulder length apart. The toes of the back foot are across from the arch of the front foot. Both knees are slightly bent. This is a very common stance in athletics. Either the left or right leg can be in the Front Stance. For example, Ward Off Right has the right front leg as Substantial. Brush Left Knee has the left front leg as Substantial.

2. <u>Back Stance</u>. The back-foot bears 90-100% of the body weight. This makes the back foot the Full or Substantial leg. The back foot is at a 45-degree angle to the front foot with the toes pointed outward. Depending on the posture, the front foot touches lightly on the toe, ball, or heel, bearing 0-10% of the body weight and is pointed straight ahead. The feet are about shoulder length apart. Both knees are slightly bent. Either the left or right leg can be in the Back Stance. For example, Raise Hands Right has the left back leg as Substantial. White Crane Spreads Wings has the right back leg as Substantial.

3. <u>Transitional Stance</u>. Both feet are almost touching at the toes while the heels remain several inches apart, similar to an open triangle. One leg will bear 90-100% of the body weight, making it the Substantial Leg. For example, this stance is used as you are making a transition from the posture Push into Single Whip.

***

The postures of Tai Chi are arranged in a sequence that shifts alternately between the Front and Back Stance. This constant shifting of the bodies weight causes the legs to work like pistons of an engine. The resulting energy is funneled to the Tan Tien as heat. Heat is the necessary catalyst to combine one's internal and external Chi.

***

MOVEMENT

Our Chi is aroused by the effects of movement, like steam from a heated pot (Soong 1995).

***

MOVEMENT:

1. Shift your weight alternately between the Substantial leg and the Insubstantial leg.
2. At least 90% of all movement requires **NO** physical exertion or force. Eliminating force reduces stress.
3. Very slow is best. Similar to a film in slow motion. This will allow you to think about what you are doing and provide time to make any necessary adjustments to eliminate stress or discomfort.

***

Tai Chi movement is founded on the doctrine of Wu- Wei or effortless action. One of the easiest ways to implement Wu-Wei is to follow the way of Nature (Chuang 4th Century BC). Move in a way that is natural to your body. It is extremely important that foot placement, the bend in the knees and the twist of the waist, all feel comfortable. The more comfortable and relaxed you are physically, the more you will be in a state of Wu-Wei.

***

The flow of Mind and external movement will set in motion a corresponding flow of Chi inside the body (Soong 1995).

***

Let the internal vapors of Chi mobilize the body. This is similar to a train using steam power to move. This is different than using muscle power (Cheng 1994).

***

Eighty percent of the movements of Tai Chi can substitute muscular exertion by applying the imagery associated with gravity, centrifugal force, momentum, and the physics involved in a coil spring.

***

Visualize the mechanics of momentum and then use your imagination to reproduce those movements as slow as possible. The Rag Doll's hips rotate and its torso and arms follow effortlessly. This will aid in the torso becoming an empty shell or Insubstantial.

***

Many Tai Chi movements are similar to the flow of a whip. The snapping of a whip is based on mechanics, not speed. It is an uncoiling action. It starts with the Gravitational force being absorbed from the ground into the Substantial foot- the handle of the whip. Then moves up the leg. The twist of the hips generates additional torque that allows the upper arms to swing and forearms to rotate. It continues through the wrist and culminates in the fingers – the tip of the whip. Each segment contributes to the uncoiling of the next. A dynamo effect in slow motion (Lee 1975).

***

When you rotate your waist in one direction with your feet firmly planted, you compress muscular energy in your lower spine. This is similar to the mechanics of a coil spring. When you unwind and go in the opposite direction, the compressed energy is released and propels the movement without the need of muscular force. Furthermore, the momentum created by the last movement can be employed to repeat the cycle.

***

A motion set in motion will remain in motion (Newton's 1st Law of Motion).

***

Imagine your upper body as an empty shell, having no bones or muscles. You don't need strength to perform any of the upper body movements. Tell your mind to direct the movements and where appropriate, utilize the concepts of momentum and gravity; not muscular force.

***

In Tai Chi, the hands and arms never move of themselves. All hand and arm movements originate from the momentum of the waist. One must absolutely not use the muscular force that is present in the hands and arms (Soong 1995).

***

Movement must be smooth and continuous (Chang 12th Century).

***

The Mind rules, the Body follows. Drive the movement with your mind, even if it's only from your imagination (Song of The Thirteen Postures (n.d.).

***

In practicing Tai Chi, the end of one posture is the beginning of the next. Each movement flows imperceptibly into the following posture. Movement is always to be slow, smooth, and soft. It should look and feel like a film in slow motion.

***

Practice slow enough so you can consciously apply the principles that define Tai Chi.

***

From beginning to end, Tai Chi movement is continuous and not broken. If adjustments are necessary, the form does allow for a brief pause at the end of the movement before going onto the next. However, do not let the mind wander. (Yang C.-F. 20th Century).

***

In Tai Chi we use stillness of the mind to control movement of the body. Let your mind be still as a mountain and your movements flow like a river (Yang C.-F. 20th Century).

***

In all movement the inner strength is rooted in the feet, developed in the legs, controlled by the waist, and expressed through the fingers (Chang 12th Century).

***

All turnings and shifting of the body weight are controlled from the waist. The movements of the limbs are an extension of the momentum generated by the waist. The waist moves and the entire body follows.

***

The source of command for all movement lies in the waist (Song of The Thirteen Postures (n.d.).

***

Movements are based on the Physical principles related to Earth and the Metaphysical concepts associated with Heaven.

Earth: Tai Chi often refers to activity from the waist down as related to the Earth and having the characteristics of being Substantial and Yang.

- <u>Gravity</u>. Feel being rooted to the earth from the waist down because of gravity.
- <u>Spring action</u> of the waist. Twisting the waist compresses energy similar to a coil spring. Unwinding releases the energy and moves the body with no exertion.
- <u>Momentum</u>. Shifting weight forward or backward requires no_exertion due to momentum. A motion set in motion stays in motion (Newton's First Law of Inertia). Many movements are the result of a previous movement that generated momentum.

<u>Heaven</u>:   Tai Chi often refers to activity from the waist up as related to Heaven and having the characteristics of being Insubstantial and Yin.

- <u>Hang from above</u>. Imagine a thread attached to the top of your head that ascends upward to Heaven. This will help keep your head, neck and spine straight.
- <u>Centrifugal Force</u>. The waist turns and the upper extremities follow like a rag doll, requiring no physical exertion. Imagine that the arms don't exist, only the fingers have substance.
- <u>Shen</u>. Imagine the Shen generated in the Tan Tien will raise like a vapor and fuel all movement above the waist. No need to use force.

RELAXATION

The Chinese term Sung means to relax, to loosen, to open, and to release tension. In Tai Chi, you Sung to create a relaxed body and mental state.

***

Relaxation is a physical state that can be controlled by the mind via "Mindfulness".

***

Wu-Wei is defined as "Unattached Action". The net effect of Wu-Wei for Tai Chi is that if you are not concerned about the results, you will be more relaxed. This will allow your body to function according to your natural inclinations, instead of "striving" to meet strict formalities. Forcing uncomfortable physical techniques will cause stress.

***

Relax the neck and position the head as if were suspended by a thread attached to the crown (Wang 18th Century AD).

***

Practice without anticipating results. Being detached from results will lead to relaxation by reducing mental and physical stress.

***

Pay close attention to relaxing the abdomen so the Chi can gather in the Tan Tien (Wang 18th Century AD).

***

To see what a relaxed abdomen looks like, seek out images of early Tai Chi Masters or those of the Buddha. They all reveal a protruding "pot belly" which is the result of a relaxed abdomen and not from overeating. Yoga emphasizes deep abdominal breathing which expands the belly outward. Tai Chi stresses relaxing the waist and sinking the breath to the lower abdomen, which creates the same effect.

***

Relaxing the abdomen can be very difficult, especially if one's vanity is a factor. Most of us have been taught that good posture involves "Chest out and stomach in". Tai Chi principles stresses just the opposite "Chest in and stomach out". Not pretty but correct. Unfortunately, a relaxed abdomen will take on the appearance of a "pot belly". Many people who are in good physical condition and not over weight, will have a small pot belly when relaxed. If you are not one of these people and have a hard time relaxing your abdomen, try the following suggestion. To get the idea of what a pot belly should look and feel like, try doing a little Tai Chi after a meal on a full stomach. It may not be comfortable and if you are full, it should be hard to hold your stomach in. Then in future practice, try to recreate the same feeling and look of a pot belly when your stomach is empty. The abdomen is the area where the Tan Tien is located, it is the pot in the belly that serves as a cauldron for enhancing and transforming Chi.

***

To generate internal energy, one must relax completely and become soft. Let go of the idea of using muscular force. Energy thrives in relaxation not tension (Wu 19th Century AD).

***

The path of studying Tai Chi must take relaxation as its training foundation (Soong 1995).

***

When the entire body is calm and relaxed, the Chi will circulate throughout the whole body (Wang 18th Century AD).

***

The easiest way to relax is to not force any given movement or strive for strict adherence to specific details related to any given posture. Force and adherence are actions that are unproductive. Instead, respond to what feels comfortable and natural. As soon as you start to feel uncomfortable, make the necessary physical adjustments to eliminate stress or tension. Even though you may physically pause a few seconds in order to readjust a posture, you are continuing the flow by mentally staying focused on the fundamental principle of "Relaxing". In other words, you can pause physically as long as you don't pause mentally. The form does allow for a brief pause at the end of the movement before going onto the next, as long as the mind doesn't wander (Yang C.-F. 20th Century).

***

THREE PHYSICAL ZONES: TOP-MIDDLE-BOTTOM

Think of a Willow tree. Its roots firmly grounded to the earth, its' trunk upright and strait, while its's branches sway easily with the winds of Heaven. Together they function as one. In Tai Chi, our bodies emulate these natural aspects of the Willow.

<u>TOP</u>

Make your spine upright and do not lean. However, holding oneself unnaturally erect will cause tension and is considered a defect (Cheng 1981).

***

Imagine that you are being hung from the crown of your head with a thread that descends down from the Heavens. This will contribute to straightening your spine and eliminate the need of muscular activity to maintain an upright torso. This is a technique to help empty the upper body of physical tension and become a vessel for the Divine.

***

Relax the torso by allowing the chest to be empty instead of protruding. Let the shoulders drop as if gravity is pulling them downward towards your fingertips. Unlock your elbows and think of your arms as rubber instead of muscle. Release the wrist so the hands can flow with the momentum of the body.

***

Think of the upper body as being Insubstantial or Yin. That means it should be totally relaxed and empty of any tension associated with muscular activity. Having an Insubstantial (Yin) upper body is one of the components necessary to combine in the Tan Tien with the opposite Substantial (Yang) of the lower body.

MIDDLE

In the middle is the Tan Tien. It is located at an area of the waist that is midpoint between front and back. It is the cauldron or melting pot for combining one's Innate internal Chi with external Natural Chi to create Shen Chi or Spirit Chi (Cheng 1994).

***

The uniting of Yin and Yang occur at the beginning and end pause of each movement. Yin and Yang unite in stillness and separate in movement. This repetitive dynamic creates a reaction that generates heat. As a result, elements of Mind and Chi are joined and become one in the Tan Tien. This combination creates spirit and eliminates anxieties (Yang C.-F. 20th Century).

***

In accordance with the philosophy of Tai Chi, all movements are from the central point or abdomen (Wen 1973).

***

The center or Tan Tien is the center of gravity of the body and the cauldron for Chi. Tan Tien literally means "field of refining vitality" (Chang 12th Century AD).

***

The Waist is the Commander of the whole body. All movements originate from here (Yang C.-Fu 20th Century AD).

***

Pay attention to the waist at all times (Song of the Thirteen Postures (n.d.).

***

In Tai Chi, the middle zone involves the Physical region of the waist and the Metaphysical spot of the Tan Tien. Focus on the middle area when turning, twisting, moving forward or back, and when pausing between movements.

***

The waist is the body's symbolic representation of the Tai Chi symbol. Where Yin/Heaven and Yang/Earth come together to create Man/Life (Tung 20th Century AD).

***

Make you waist soft as though it is absolutely without bone, totally loosened and relaxed (Yang C.-F. 20th Century).

***

The area of the waist contains the Tan Tien and the Pelvic Girdle. Visualize the Pelvic Girdle as a powerful gear that rotates the waist.

***

With the lower abdomen completely loosened, the Chi will ascend on its own (Song of the Thirteen Postures (n.d.).

***

BOTTOM

Heaviness is the foundation for lightness. When the legs and feet are attached to the ground with heaviness (Substantial), the upper body will feel secure and free to be light and empty (Insubstantial).

***

From the waist down the legs act like mechanical pistons, generating energy that is converted to heat in the Tan Tien. The shifting back and forth of bodily weight on slightly bent knees requires the leg muscles, especially the thighs, to generate a level of tension. This is normal. The bottom halve of the body is full of tension (not tightness) while the top halve of the body is empty of tension. The bottom halve is Substantial (Full-Positive-Yang) and the top halve is Insubstantial (Empty-Negative-Yin). When these two opposite conditions meet in the center (Tan Tien), there is a reaction (Lao Tzu 5th Century AD). Positive electrons meet Negative electrons and heat is the result. It's this heat that fuses internal and external Chi to create Shen.

***

There is a difference between muscle tension and muscle tightness (Lee 1975).

***

You take up energy from the earth through your feet.

***

After every movement the body must be relaxed and the rootedness of the feet must be reestablished.

***

Find your footing first.

***

Imagine being rooted to the earth from the waist down.

***

Be centered, rooted, and still as a mountain (Chang 12th Century). As you practice, pause long enough to establish being balanced, stable, and calm.

***

Don't be misled by the phrase "Continuous motion". It's ok to pause for a few seconds between postures. "Continuous motion" means to continue the exercise until you have completed all the postures that make up the sequence of your Form. The sequence of the Form was designed to generate heat by the constant shifting of body weight from Substantial (Yang) to Insubstantial (Yin).

***

MENTAL

Early Chinese text suggested that a person's Mind can be made to suffuse the body as a fluid like essence. The concept of Chi is often used in the context of being a fluid like entity that can embody consciousness (Yang C.-F. 2005). This idea seems logical, if you accept the theory that Chi is in all things, both tangible and intangible.

***

At every moment, attention has to be paid to the mind (Wu 19th Century AD).

***

Intent of the mind can be used to create movement or stillness.

***

Just the process of thinking will combine Consciousness with Chi in the Tan Tien. You may ask, what does this mean? Just having the thought that your mind can visit the Tan Tien to gather existing Chi, will cause it to happen. You don't have to force it, just think of it frequently. Consciousness will gather the Chi automatically. This is an example of getting results without having to do anything but initiate the process. This is Wu-Wei or doing by not doing (Yang C.-F. 20th Century AD).

***

It is necessary to maintain a calm mind (Li 19thCentury AD).

***

Be master of your mind, rather than mastered by your mind (Buddha (ed.)1993).

***

Mental thoughts can trigger physical changes. You're not hungry but you start salivating after seeing a commercial of your favorite food. Using one's imagination to implement many of the techniques associated with Tai Chi is a fundamental concept.

***

Cultivate peace of mind. Peace of mind produces right thought. Right thought produces right action (Buddha (ed.) 1993).

***

When engaging the mind in "Mindfulness" while practicing, you are distracting the Ego from its' constraints. Thus, allowing the body to respond to its natural inclinations.

***

The Mind wanders wherever pleasure, desire, or lust leads it, but during Tai Chi practice it can be tamed and guided with Mindfulness (Buddha (ed.) 1993).

***

Practicing Tai Chi requires the mind to focus on various principles and techniques. This requires "Mindfulness".

***

In addition to providing the physical benefits related to exercise, Tai Chi is also highly recommended as a form of mental relaxation or Meditation.

***

Meditation is not some type of esoteric trance that takes years to learn. It is a simple mental exercise that encourages you to focus on something other than the stress generated by Life's daily concerns.

***

The purpose of Meditation is to produce a relaxed and tranquil mind by eliminating the constant stream of jumbled and negative thoughts that cause stress. Five to Fifteen minutes of Meditation does the same thing for your mind that a nap does for your body.

It allows your system to rest and recharge.

***

Tai Chi can be a Meditation when performed with "Mindfulness". Mindfulness means to concentrate strictly on the activity you are engaged in, moment by moment.

***

When practicing Tai Chi, meditate on what you are doing. There are plenty of mechanics and concepts you can focus on at any given moment. Concentrate solely on the particulars of the posture or movement you are performing. This is performing an activity with "Mindfulness".

***

At every moment, attention has to be paid to the Mind (Wu 19th Century).

***

It is natural for your mind to wander to everyday thoughts such as: "What am I having for dinner? Did I lock the car? Are the kids alright? Etc." Each time you find your mind wandering, don't get frustrated (that causes stress), just return to concentrating on what you are doing. Tell yourself you'll address those issues when you're done with Tai Chi. Some days your mind will wander more than others. Regardless, learn not to get frustrated when your mind does wander. This strategy will allow you to be in a Meditative state most of the time while practicing Tai Chi. True meditation does not require perfection. Striving for perfection indicates an attachment to the action. That is not Wu Wei.

***

Jesus said "Will all your worries add a single moment to your life?" (Matthew 6:27).

***

CENTRAL EQUILIBRIUM

Tai Chi is an exercise that requires balance which is based on centering physically. Central Equilibrium results in balance, and balance is the key to graceful movement. Good physical balance in our daily lives is one of the most important benefits of Tai Chi. Accidental falls can be avoided with improved balance.

***

In every movement during practice, one must maintain the condition of Central Equilibrium (Liang 21st Century).

***

Central Equilibrium is accomplished by balancing on one leg that has the full weight, while remaining comfortable and relaxed. The weight must be stable and rooted before slowly transferred to the opposite leg. This must be accomplished with a smooth transition while remaining upright and not leaning in any direction (Soong 1995).

***

Centering physically allows the waist to revolve in a balanced and fluid manner. Without Central Equilibrium nothing else will work correctly. That is how relevant it is. With a balanced lower body, the upper body can fully relax.

***

In Tai Chi, Central Equilibrium is both a physical and mental state of being which can be achieved in various ways. The simplest explanation is to keep the body vertical and perpendicular to the ground, while transitioning from one posture to the next. To aid in establishing Central Equilibrium, bend your knees and lowery your center of gravity to increase your physical awareness and stability. Stabilizing the center should not involve any form of physical tension. In practicing Tai Chi, the goal is to maintain Central Equilibrium as we shift alternately between the Substantial and Insubstantial leg.

***

Central Equilibrium also has a philosophical concept. It is about awareness and Life Style. Mentally, we can enhance our physical balance by adopting an attitude towards life that integrates and reconciles opposites, rather than excluding one from the other. When we are at peace with ourselves, the mind will be relaxed and tranquil which will aid in balancing the body and enhancing Central Equilibrium.

***

By maintaining stability via Central Equilibrium during practice, you learn not to lean. An upright, stable body works constructively with gravity to assist with balance, much more efficiently than slumping or leaning. Leaning creates muscular tension to avoid falling towards the lean.

***

The upright body must be stable and comfortable (Wu 19th Century).

***

YIN / YANG

This section on Yin/Yang is very basic and only relates to its association with Tai Chi. It is far from complete and the reader can explore a more in-depth explanation on their own.

***

The *Tai Chi Chuan Treatise* tells us that Yin and Yang is the mother of Tai Chi. The mutual cooperation of Yin and Yang is precisely what makes up the understanding of energy (Chang 12th Century).

***

This form of exercise is named Tai Chi because its concepts are based on the power and dynamics of the Yin/Yang principles. While performing a movement, Yin separates from Yang but at the end of the movement Yin reunites with Yang and creates energy (Wen 1973). Tai Chi uses this energy to produce heat in the Tan Tien which combines Internal Innate Chi with External Nature chi. The result is Shen Chi that is a vapor like essence that permeates the body to be used or stored.

***

Yin/Yang can be subdivided into additional Yin/Yang aspects. For example, the lower body is always Yang but is subdivided into one leg being Yin (empty, insubstantial, negative) and the other leg being Yang (full, substantial, positive). Likewise, the upper body is Yin but separated into a Yin arm and a Yang arm. Moreover, the subdivisions of the arms and legs are constantly alternating between Yin and Yang as the body weight is shifted from one leg to the other. This constant changing from positive to negative is what generates energy. This energy is converted to heat.

***

Yin/Yang are two complementary forces that make up all aspects of life. Both are said to proceed from the Divine (Lao Tzu 5th Century BC).

***

Yin/Yang are opposite principles that interact in a complementary manner.

***

Yin/Yang are two opposite parts. When united, they become whole or complete. It is "Duality" merging into "Oneness".

***

When separate; Yin is passive, empty, insubstantial, negative; and Yang is active, full, substantial, positive. When they join in the Tan Tien, they create energy or heat. Similar to the concept of electricity being generated when negative and positive electrons come together.

***

When you practice Tai Chi, you learn to relax your upper body so it becomes Yin, while allowing your lower body to become Yang, more solid, and heavy.

***

In Tai Chi, the body is divided according to Yin/Yang categories. The upper body corresponds to Yin, while the lower body is rooted in Yang. The body's center (Tan Tien) is where they unite.

***

TAN TIEN

The center of gravity in the human body is the Tan Tien. It is also considered the "Psychic Center". It is located about 2 inches below the navel and midway between the front and back of the body (Wen 1973).

***

All movements originate from the Tan Tien. The rotation of the pelvic girdle causes outward movement of Chi to the arms and legs (Wu 19th Century AD).

***

The whole body is filled with Chi. The Tan Tien is where the mind gathers the Chi. The reaction caused by the changes of Yin and Yang generates heat in the Tan Tien. The heat combines one's internal and external Chi into Shen, then transforms it into an enriched vapor. The vapor can be stored in stillness or activated for motion (Wang T.-Y. 15th Century AD).

***

From the breath, man draws the invisible, ungraspable force of the Universe for compounding the elixir in the Tan Tien to create Shen/Spirit (Wen 1973).

***

The Tan Tien is the main tool for enriching the Chi. Our hearts pump blood and the Tan Tien pumps Chi.

***

Let the whole body relax and center the mind on the Tan Tien. The special ability of Tai Chi is its ability to gather the Chi in the Tan Tien (Cheng 1981).

PRACTICE

How much time you spend practicing Tai Chi will vary, depending on how much time you spend doing other types of exercise or activities. You should attempt to spend a minimum of about 5-15 minutes a session, 4-5 times a week. Once or twice a day is ideal but even a few minutes a day will produce many of the benefits.

***

A day's effort gives a day's results. A year's effort gives a year's results.

***

Participants should strive for daily practice and not be concerned about perfection of performance. Correctness (not perfection) will develop when muscle memory can assist while performing the sequence. Practicing the FORM from memorization, frees the mind to focus on the fundamental mechanics and principles of Tai Chi.

***

The Yin/Yang concept embraces the reality that every time you practice, there will be strong points and weak points to your Form. It's the things you've incorporated and the things you didn't incorporate that creates the totality of your practice.

***

It is nearly impossible to employ all of the suggested techniques at any one given moment of practice. The Yin/Yang concept allows for the reality that you will vacillate among and between the various key points during practice.

***

Develop confidence in your own style of practicing Tai Chi. Age, body type, level of fitness, medical factors, etc., are all variables of what will determine your style of practice. Everyone has their own unique style, just like their fingerprint.

***

Postures and movement should be modified to feel comfortable and natural to your particular body type and fitness. Nothing should feel stressed or uncomfortable. Initially, you may feel some discomfort from using muscles you are not use to using, but your body will adapt after a few sessions. How you perform the postures may change over time, depending on your understanding and internalization of the fundamentals.

***

Practicing Tai Chi is an ongoing process that will continue to evolve and change depending on what aspect is being focused on. Consequently, it is a mistake to be concerned about what you look like or how well you perform the sequence.

***

Focus on the fundamental mechanics of proper body alignment but do not be overly concerned about exact foot/hand placement and related movements. They vary greatly among the different styles of Tai Chi and who is performing them.

***

As one's practice gradually becomes refined, one's concentration of external movement will be reduced and one's concentration of internal movement will be increased (Cheng 1994).

***

In time, one will gradually become more intimate with the internal principles of the art (Chang 12th Century AD).

***

When finished with practice, don't cool off immediately by washing or drinking water. This will cause a stagnation of the

Chi that has been activated by the heat generated from exercise. Allow your body a few minutes to absorb the benefits created by practicing Tai Chi (Cheng 1999).

***

Some movements will be smooth and satisfactory while others may be rough and weak. Furthermore, different days may yield different results for different postures. When it comes to reflecting on your performance, think in terms of percentages as the professional athletes do. If you feel comfortable about how 70% of your practice went, you are doing great! No need to be perfect. Seeking perfection will only lead to stress. The important thing is to remain steadfast in your daily practice.

***

On the days you just don't feel like practicing, you can still stay connected to Tai Chi by pursuing other venues. You can read, research, meditate, or get on the Web and watch Tai Chi videos. Also, just standing and shifting your weight from one leg to the other for a few seconds is better than doing nothing. Sometimes this simple action can be a catalyst and motivate you to do a little more.

***

Tai Chi Master, Lu Zi-Jian lived to be 118 (1893-2012). When asked what his secret to longevity was, he said: Keep moving and do something every day of your life (Waysun 1990).

***

As you practice and progress, remain humble to the unfathomable vastness of this unexplainable phenomena (Yang C.-F. 20th Century AD.). The Tai Chi Classic's adage "Flow like a powerful river" suggest that our internal Chi will move with power through the pathways of our body. Furthermore, it is also interpreted to remind us that as a river eventually flows and unites into the massiveness of the sea, we should let our spirit flow and merge into the vastness of the Divine.

***

When practicing, allow the mind to visit the Tan Tien. Do not forget to do this, but do not coerce it. The Chi will automatically spread through the body. You cannot force it; it will happen naturally. Have faith (Cheng 1994).

***

Master Li I-Yu, author of *Five Character Secret,* was asked what were his favorite postures and he replied "Practicing only Grasps the Sparrows Tail will provide all the benefits associated with Tai Chi." (Li p. 71) The combination of Postures Ward Off, Pull Back, Press, and Push; are often referred to as one posture called Grasp The Sparrow's Tail.

***

Key points to observe when practicing Tai Chi as generalized from the Tai Chi Classics:

1. Form and technique are the least important aspects of Tai Chi. Perseverance is the priority.

2. Relax. Use the least amount of muscular force possible. Let the mechanics of physics do the work.

3. Imagine a thread suspending the head from above. Don't let the head tilt in any direction.

4. Your stance should be comfortable and able to move easily in any direction.

5. Keep the neck and spine straight. Do not to lean.

6. The weight on your legs should constantly be shifting from Substantial to Insubstantial.

7. Let your waist revolve smoothly, creating momentum that moves the arms and hands.

8. Relax the Mind by focusing on what you are doing.

"Mindfulness".

9. Breath naturally. Don't create stress by trying to control it.

10. Move slow enough so you can apply the appropriate mental and physical concepts.

It is nearly impossible to employ all of the above at any one given moment. The Yin/Yang concept allows for the reality that you will vacillate among and between the various key points during practice.

***

KEEP IT SIMPLE

Out of clutter, find simplicity (Einstein 1994).

***

Most successful coaches and athletes will tell you that their success is based on focusing on the fundamentals and not getting distracted by a flood of extraneous options and details. Stick to the few fundamentals that make up the instructional core of the Tai Chi Classics.

***

One of the most renowned instructional Tai Chi Classics is the Song of Thirteen Postures. It is only 140 Chinese characters.

***

Bruce Lee stressed it didn't make a difference how you performed a move, just do it. A punch is a punch and a kick is a kick (Lee. 1975).

***

In the beginner's mind there are many possibilities, but in the expert's mind there are few (Suzuki 1994).

***

Similar to any large body of information, you have to sift out the facts from the fluff.

***

With so many prolific writers and resources available, the study of Tai Chi can easily become an over whelming and endless pursuit. Refine your efforts to the basic. Forgo the techniques that promise mystical feats of extraordinary power or accomplishments. There have been more than a few Tai Chi experts who performed amazing acts, only later to be revealed as fakes and charlatans.

***

There are many exciting tangents and layers to discover which will certainly enrich your understanding of this fascinating art. However, there is no substitute for spending a few minutes practicing Tai Chi every day while focusing on the basic suggestions offered by the Masters found in the Tai Chi Classics.

***

Millions of people who have never read a Tai Chi book or seen a video have benefited from the practice of Tai Chi for over 2000 years by simply adhering to a few fundamentals taught by a competent instructor.

***

Most of the Tai Chi books by current authors can exceed several hundred pages. In contrast, the instructional articles found in the Tai Chi Classics are very brief and usually less than one page. For example, Yang Cheng Fu's Ten Essential Points is roughly only 444 words long.

***

These 10 Points express all of the principles necessary to become proficient at practice and receive all the benefits associated with Tai Chi.

***

Following are the Ten Essential Points of Yang Chen Fu from his book: *APPLICATION METHODS OF TAIIQUAN* (Yang C.-F. 20th Century).

1. Elevate the crown and lift the spirit. The head should be upright so the Shen or (spirit) can reach the top of your head.

2. Contain the chest, expand the back. The chest is slightly sunken so that the chi can sink to the Tan Tien,

3. Sung (Relax) your waist. The waist is the commander in charge of your whole body. If you can relax your waist then your legs will have the power and your lower parts will be stable and strong.

4. Understand the difference between insubstantial and substantial. This is one of the very first things you will learn in Tai Chi. If the weight is on the right leg, then the right leg is substantial and the left leg is insubstantial. When these can be separated and consciously acknowledged, you will be able to turn lightly without using any tension or stress.

5. Sink the shoulders and drop down the elbows. Your shoulders should be completely relaxed downward and open to the sides. Sink the elbows. This means that your elbows move downward and stay relaxed. If you raise the elbows the shoulders also go up. Keeping the shoulders and elbows down gives your body internal power.

6. Use the mind and not force. When practicing Tai Chi, relax your whole body.

7. Coordinate the upper and lower body. The classics tell us that "the motion should be rooted in the feet, released through the legs, controlled by the waist and manifested through the fingers." The whole body moves as one unit, nothing broken or disconnected between upper and lower body.

8. Internal and external coordinate. Relaxing into the movements sends the energy and blood out to the limbs, now the whole body is nourished, regulating blood pressure, relaxing the soft tissues and veins/arteries and calming the entire nervous system. The mind and body are now working together as we practice our form.

9. Continuity without breakage. From beginning to end, Tai Chi movement is continuous and not broken. After each movement it starts again, circulating without any end. The form does allow for a brief rest at the end of the movement before going onto the

next.

10. Seek stillness within movement. Tai Chi is known as a moving meditation. In Tai Chi we use stillness to control movement. Even though we are moving, there is still stillness. It is good to practice your form slowly, with calmness and awareness. We can see that although the body moves as one unit, it does not all move at the same time.

***

Six fundamental concepts for practicing Tai Chi:

The various postures, movements, and fundamentals of Tai Chi emphasize specific chapters of the I-Ching. They were design as a reminder of how the practitioner should interact with others on a daily basis. The I-Ching passages below correspond to six basic concepts of Tai Chi (I-CHING 9th Century BC).

1. Acknowledge Tai Chi as a moving prayer. Do not be concerned about Form. Spirit is the priority.

I-CHING # 40: Forgive mistakes and pardon wrongs.

2. The Mind leads all movements and the body follows.

I-CHING # 57: What is Willed is carried out in action.

3. From the waist up, be flexible. Momentum moves the arms and hands.

I-CHING: #22: Flexibility comes forth to embellish firmness.

4. At the waist be centered. Revolve the waist like a wheel.

I-CHING #51: Remain balanced and calm in the center.

5. From the waist down be firm. Shift from substantial to insubstantial.

I-CHING #31: Flexibility comes from above "Heaven" and firmness comes from below "Earth".

6. Do not lean. Spine and head are upright.

I-Ching #19: Being up right and true is the way to Heaven.

***

BEGINNER'S BASICS

Learn one basic Tai Chi routine (called a Form), and stick with it.
***

The easiest style and most commonly taught is the Yang Style. The Yang style can have as many as 3 sections with a total of 107 postures. However, the most practiced is the short Yang style made popular by Cheng Man Ching. The short Yang routine is composed of approximately 37 postures.
***

The best strategy for a novice is to begin by learning only the first section. The first section is often known as the Original Thirteen. It has 13-18 postures, depending on the school or style of Tai Chi. Keep in mind, it's not how many postures you perform, but how well you perform them with Mindfulness.
***

Concentrate on memorizing just the Original Thirteen or first section. You want to be able to practice the postures, without thinking about what the next movement is. It needs to become automatic or second nature. That will allow you to focus on the various mechanics and philosophy that accompanies each posture. Once you have mastered the first section, you can move on to the other sections. However, you only need to practice the Original Thirteen or first section to receive all of Tai Chi's benefits.
***

A good strategy for leaning the first section is to get a basic book that explains the postures and closely reflects the Original Thirteen sequence. Again, limit yourself to the shortest routine possible. Then, incorporate the teachings from the Tai Chi Classics into your practice.
***

Also, watch You-Tube videos of people in your age bracket. This will give you a realistic impression of what Tai Chi may look like for someone like yourself. If you're not 18 years old and a gymnast, don't expect your Form to look like the returning National Tai Chi Champion of Taiwan. You may be surprised how bland and unpretentious Tai Chi can look when done correctly by ordinary citizens. The reason for this is because the practitioner has successfully internalized the fundamentals and is not preoccupied by what the external Form looks like. Below are a few videos from the web of Tai Chi performed by both Masters and students.
***

1. www. Heaven, Earth, Man Taijiquan Section One (3:09 minutes)
2. www. Taiji For Meditation, Section One-Heaven, Earth, Man Taijiquan (2:42 minutes)
3. www. Yang Family Tai Chi Long Form First Section (3:19 minutes)
4. www. Chen Man Ching Disciple of Yang Chen (4:40 minutes)
5. www. Traditional Yang Style Long Form Taijiquan First Part (5:08 min.)
6. www.Yang Jwing-Ming. "Yang Tai Chi for Beginners" (3:52 minutes)
7. www. Wang Qing Yu-Traditional Yang Tai Chi Chuan (4:46 minutes)

***

For a detailed explanation of how to perform 95% of the Forms presented in the first section of the Yang style, watch the 6 short videos produced by LIVING MOMENTS TAI CHI with instructor Angus Clark. Each video is separate and last 6-7 minutes. Get on the internet and type each title to see that specific Form/movement.
Tai Chi Form 1 Beginning.
Tai Chi Form 2 Ward off left & ward off right.
Tai Chi Form 3 Roll back, press, & push.
Tai Chi Form 4 Single whip.

Tai Chi Form 5 Lifting hands, shoulder stroke, white crane spreads wings.

Tai Chi Form 6 Brush left knee & push, play guitar (raise hands left), brush left knee & push

***

When learning from a book or video, stick to the suggestions presented in the chapter PERSONAL STYLE. It's important to remember that it is not necessary to focus on external formalities, such as exact foot or hand placement. Instead, pay attention to the philosophical and spiritual elements that will lead to the true benefits that Tai Chi has to offer.

***

Taking a Tai Chi class by a competent teacher can also be a good idea. A knowledgeable instructor will adhere to the principles of the Tai Chi Classics. Especially the concept: "Do not force the body into uncomfortable or stress provoking postures". How can exact foot or hand placement be a factor, if there are so many variations depending on the school or style of Tai Chi? Persistence and the fundamental principles of the Tai Chi Classics are the only true requirements for success.

***

STRATEGIES FOR SENIORS

I'm using the term Seniors as a method to target a few additional strategies to apply in the pursuit of Tai Chi. I am not stereotyping an age-related phenomenon that can easily miscommunicate who a person is. How you feel physically and mentally can often fluctuate week from week, relative to a variety of factors that infringe upon your life. Regardless, if you feel like a Senior sometimes, this chapter may be helpful.

***

There are a few basic tips that everyone can benefit from. How you approach these tips depends on your age, overall health, and time constraints. Just like Tai Chi, tailor these suggestions to your individual needs. Don't hesitate to hold on to something for support, lay on the bed (instead of the floor), or modify routines to fit your abilities. Be creative. If you condense these activities to a few minutes, they will be easy to implement into a busy life.

***

1. BEFORE SLEEP. Prepare for tomorrow by getting a good night's rest. This is more involved than just getting between the sheets and calling it a night. It should begin with not having a belly full of food. A light snack that doesn't push against the Tan Tien is fine, but nothing heavy enough to make you feel uncomfortable before your bed-time routine. What routine? Read on.

Unless you just completed some type of physical exercise that stretched muscles and unlocked joints, you should do something that will relax your body. A few minutes of Tai Chi, Qi Gong, Yoga, or any type of stretching, should be enough to relieve the physical stress that your body accumulated over the last few hours of the day. Design your own routine. Keep it simple and short, but do something. Anything is better than nothing!

***

After you reduced physical tension with a little stretching, freshen up. Take a shower, bath, or wash thoroughly. Floss and Brush your teeth. You want to feel clean all over. An age-old proverb states: "Cleanliness is next to Godliness". It simply means that cleaning your body is symbolic of aspiring towards spiritual virtue. You can freshen up first; then stretch. It doesn't make a difference what the sequence is, just try to do them 5 – 7 times a week.

The idea is to prepare yourself for an 8-hour event. Approach sleep for what it is: an experience into another reality.

The better you prepare for sleep, the better you will feel when you awake.

***

2. AFTER SLEEP. You have just laid dormant for several hours. You need to warm up your body. Similar to how athletes warm up before competition, you need to prepare for what the new day will bring. Again, it is best to start with a few gentle stretches. Try to work out the morning kinks that sleep can leave behind. A few "knee bends" and "toe touches", along with various "twist" can be enough to get you going. Hold on to something, if balance is an issue. If your mobility is limited, improvise. There are plenty of ideas available on the web. Tailor your routine to something that is easy enough to do without getting discouraged. Keeping it short to a few minutes will help. Next, wash the sand out of your eyes. Also, rinsing with a little mouth wash will help liven you up.

***

Now that you have taken care of the outside of your body, do something for the inside. After several hours of not drinking any liquids during sleep, your body will be dehydrated. The best thing you can do first thing in the morning is to have something warm to drink. Enjoy a hot cup of coffee, tea, lemon water, or whatever you find tasteful and relaxing. A cool glass of juice or water is fine, but a warm liquid inside your system will help activate the core of your being.

***

3. DURING THE DAY. In between your normal daily activities, your body is going to absorb stress. Just 1-3 minutes of stretching, twisting, bending, etc., can do wonders to unlock and release accumulated tension. Again, frequency depends on how your body responds to stress. Usually, the older you are the quicker your body will tighten up, and the more you have to address it.

***

Do your joints creak, pop, and moan when you stretch? If they do, then you should understand the importance of frequent stretching. You can use the same mini routine for relieving night, morning, and afternoon stress. You don't have to do a lot, but you should do something. As we grow older, our bodies become like aging vehicles. It takes a little longer to warm up and if it sits too long, rust will start to take its toll. Keeping the joints and spine loose and lubricated helps reduce the negative impact of arthritis and other age-related symptoms.

***

Needless to say, what you eat and drink during the day will affect your feeling of well-being. Moderation is the key. Eat for fuel 80% of the time and eat less for fun. No donuts are best, but 1 is better than 2. No need to deprive yourself of anything, just don't overeat. Your body functions much more efficiently when it is not bogged down with a full belly.

***

Encouraging spiritual growth is a basic doctrine of Tai Chi. Take a minute and count your blessings. Pray. Give thanks for what you have. Do this often and remind yourself the body is a living Temple for the Divine. Furthermore, stay spiritually centered by exhibiting compassionate behavior towards all things, including yourself.

***

No need to be a slave to any type of regiment, just try to do the right thing most of the time. Attempt to adhere to a weekly plan that reflects good habits 80% of the time. It helps to keep a weekly or monthly chart that indicates how often you exercise, reflects your eating habits and monitors your weight.

***

The above suggestions are based on the Tai Chi concepts of allowing your Chi to flow by keeping your muscles relaxed, your mind moving, and your spirit active. Remember, you want to employ the concepts of Tai Chi not only when you are practicing, but throughout your life. This philosophy will contribute greatly to receiving the benefits associated with Tai Chi.

***

Along with practicing Tai Chi, you should include as much variation into your weekly fitness goals as possible. Adhering to only one form of exercise can become boring and limited. You should include frequent walks, light weights, range of motion movements, aerobics, yoga, outside activities, etc. The is no limit to the list for achieving good health.

***

ORIGINAL THIRTEEN

Tai Chi initially consisted of only 13 postures related to specific Trigrams and their significance, as connotated in the I-Ching. Eventually other styles were developed incorporating as many as 109 postures. However, most styles still start by performing the Original Thirteen movements as their first section. Second and Third sections involve repeating the postures of the Original 13 along with adding several new movements. The purpose for expanding the Original 13 was to provide a longer exercise routine. However, The Yang style was later condensed by Chen Man Cheng to 37 postures to encourage more people to practice Tai Chi.

***

Each of the Original Thirteen Tai Chi movements were designed to remind the practitioner of the Philosophical and Spiritual foundations of the I CHING. Along with being a physical and mental exercise, it is also meant to be practiced as a symbolic form of prayer that acknowledges the omnipresence of the Divine.

****

There is some variation among authors concerning what I CHING Trigrams best corresponds to each of the Original Thirteen postures. However, they all agree that Tai Chi has its' origin in the spiritual roots of the I CHING. The idea is to bring these spiritual axioms to life by integrating them into our daily lives.

***

Trigrams are a cryptographic code used as ciphers to illuminate philosophical and spiritual phenomena as presented in the I CHING. A Trigram is a graphic symbol composed of 3 horizontal lines that can be either complete, broken, or a combination of each. There is a total of 64 in the I CHING. Below are 8 examples.

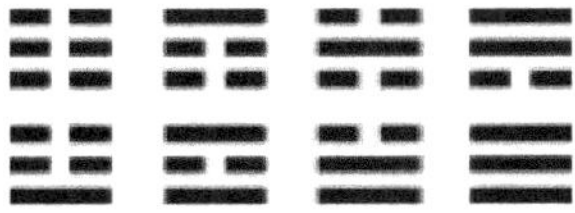

***

Following are the Original Thirteen Forms. The spiritual phrases expressed, represent the meaning of the Trigrams they are linked to in the I Ching. The relationships and interpretations are from Stuart Olson's book *T'AI CHI ACCORDING TO THE I CHING* (Olson 2002).

0. MEDITATIVE MOMENT:

One senses that the body no longer exists and the wise person's thoughts do not go beyond this moment. When the mind rest in the state of nothingness, look at the internal aspects.

1.   *HOMAGE TO HEAVEN:*

Heaven is full of strength and the wise persons draws on this strength unceasingly. The greatness of a wise person's character is to endure everything.

2.   *WARD OFF:*

To merge with the Divine. All things originate from it. Live in harmony with the Spirit. This is what benefits the upright and true.

3.   *PULL BACK:*

Once a decision is made, it is done and you are transported to a higher level of responsibility. Follow   and find the Lord. What is willed is carried out in action.

4.   *PRESS:*

The soul is always in danger of stagnation. Like water, it must flow from the source and be transformed. Go through dangerous straits without losing your faith.

5.   *PUSH:*

It is advantages to be firm and correct. Clinging to what is Right, develops the world.

6. *SINGLE WHIP:*

Be joyous together and have empathy for those who suffer. This is the way to accord with Heaven and respond to humanity. Joy shows the pleasure of inward harmony.

7.   *RAISE HANDS:*

Startling thunder brings fear but does not cause loss of scared devotion.

8.   *SHOULDER STROKE:*

When action and stillness do not miss their timing, the path is Illuminated. The wise person weights all things and makes them equal and right.

9.   *WHITE CRANE SPREADS WINGS:*

When the wise person discovers what is correct, they will follow it. When they discover errors, they correct them.

10.   *BRUSH LEFT KNEE:*

As you move forward in Life, act with the strength of metal. The wise person is constantly reexamining themselves and so forever improves upon their nature.

11.   *DEFLECT DOWNWARD, PARRY, AND PUNCH:*

The wise person's heart is limitless. They are boundless in both support and protection of others.

12.   *APPARENT CLOSURE:*

The wise person restrains themselves in order to avoid dangers. They seek neither praise nor gain.

13.   *CROSS HANDS:*

Be stable, centered, and find calmness in the Divine. A Men.

***

The ultimate purpose of Tai Chi is to provide us with wisdom and insights that we can apply to life. If we cannot do that, then it doesn't matter how well we perform the movements and postures. True Tai Chi must be lived (Lin 1964).

***

The Tai Chi Classics state to develop one's Spiritual Being is the real contribution of Tai Chi (Waysun 1990).

THE EVOLUTION OF TAI CHI

Following is a brief explanation and time line of the evolution of the exercise known as Tai Chi Chuan, commonly referred to as Tai Chi in Western practice.

***

To begin with, the concept of "God" has over 100 different names, depending on the culture it is associated with. To list just a few; there is Yahweh, Lord, Father in Heaven, Shiva, Buddha, Great Spirit, Allah, the Divine, Cosmic Consciousness, etc. In Taoism, Tai Chi means the Grand Ultimate. Roughly, this is the Chinese equivalent to the concept of God.

***

The concepts related to the term Tai Chi first appears in a document called the I CHING. It was written around 800 BC. It is considered one of the world's greatest Philosophical and Spiritual books. It emphasizes that the Divine exists within all things. The I-CHING #1 states: Vast indeed is the scope of the greatness of the Creative Basis. All things and all beings originate from it (I-CHING 9th Century BC).

***

The I CHING inspired the document *The Yellow Emperor's Classic of Internal Medicine.* It was written around 300 BC. It developed a system of mental & physical exercises that would help heal & energize the internal organs. The exercises were called Qi Gong. The concept was to preserve the physical body because it serves as a temple for the Divine.

***

Somewhere around 100 AD., *The Twelve Nerve Exercises* were developed. They integrated concepts of Acupuncture to existing Qi Gong exercises. The exercises stressed that blocked nerves create various problems.

***

Approximately 500 AD., *The Eight Directional Exercises* came into practice. Qi Gong movements were performed while aligning the body to the magnetic poles of the earth to "recharge" one's electrical forces.

***

Also, around 500 AD., an unnamed woman in the Court of King Gou Jian was recorded to be the first person to incorporate individual internal exercises into a continuous flow known as Nei Chia, the predecessor to Tai Chi.

***

A Taoist Monk, Chang San Feng is credited as the founder of Tai Chi around 1250 AD. He combined the best parts of all the preceding Internal Medicine Strategies and Qi Gong Exercises into one continuous flow of sequential movement called Tai Chi Chuan. In the beginning, Tai Chi had only 13 postures, known as the *Original Thirteen*. They were a combination of 8 hand movements and 5-foot movements, as depicted in the Eight Trigrams from the I-Ching, symbolizing GOD's presence and action in all things.

***

MY PATH TO TAI CHI

I was raised in Pittsburgh's inner city where frequent fist fights were part of growing up. I learned the basic skills of street fighting at an early age. An ability to defend yourself and a reputation of "Toughness" was a necessity for survival in our neighborhood. As a young adult, I continued to improve my pugilistic skills through strength training, boxing, collegiate wrestling, and a variety of martial arts.

***

I was fortunate never to be seriously hurt in any of my 20 plus street fights. My first occurred when I was in the third grade and the last happened towards the end of my senior year at college. Many of my fights were related to gangs I was part of and others were just a result of the circumstances I found myself in.

***

In my late 20's I had an epiphany and realize that I could grow beyond an Ego that function from a perspective that had been molded on aggression and self-righteousness. Instead of adhering to a mind set of "I'm right and you're wrong", I began to internalize the concept of "Oneness". The belief that all things are connected and share the same Divine source of creation. This led to an interest in Eastern Philosophy and Meditation. I took a Yoga class and was impressed with the immediate benefits I experienced physically, mentally, and spiritually.

During this same period, I was also studying Shotokan Karate. One day at the Dojo, a neighbor of mine who was a Police Officer and a 2nd Degree Black Belt, approached me while we I was practicing some hand hardening drills. I was punching into a bucket of sand. He knew I was an Art teacher and interested in Yoga. He said "Why do you want to toughen your hands, you're an artist. This Hard style of Karate may not be the best Martial Art for you. You should check out Tai Chi. It is a Soft style of Kung Fu and doesn't involve the traditional hard-core training of Karate." I went to the Tai Chi instructor he suggested and observed a class. The following week I started studying with Master Kim Yo Chou. A few years later, Master Chou asked me to assist him with one of his classes. After six months, he suggested that I continue teaching the class on my own. That was the beginning of my commitment to teaching Tai Chi.

***

A PERSONAL TRIBUTE

Most people persist to engage in specific exercises, diets, or other healthful activities because they like the results. I have continued to practice Tai Chi for over 45 years because of the ongoing benefits I experience.

For example, over the years I have encountered a lot of potential incidences that could have ended with a major injury or similar disaster. For instance, instead of falling from a misstep or trip, I have been able to keep my balance without stumbling. Improved balance is a product of Tai Chi. Quick reflexes has also been another obvious improvement. Occasionally I have bumped objects off a shelf and caught them without a conscious effort or looking. These are preventive actions that occur frequently. Furthermore, the enhanced Chi that results from practice has helped me endure and recover from a host of medical concerns. This includes everything from being able to relax in the Dentist's chair to recovering from major surgery. Perhaps most important are the situations that can only be explained as Divine Intervention. Following are several personal stories that highlight the impact of Tai Chi in my life.

***

Sometime in the Spring of 1978, I was at the children's play section at the local park. I was sitting on the grass watching my 5-year son enjoying himself on the swings. In the distant, I heard an argument escalating between a group of men and women. I discreetly turned my head to see what the raucous was about. Thirty yards away, I saw two teenage girls walking away from three tall men who appeared to be "Tough Guys". The men had beer bottles in their hands and were yelling profanities at the young women as they were leaving. I turned my focus back to my son who was still on the swing. I did not want to draw any attention to myself. Within seconds, I saw the men walking in my direction. The leader, who was shirtless, except for a leather vest that revealed a tattooed chest, appeared to be hiding something in his hand. After he took a few more steps, it became obvious he was holding a large knife and was coming directly towards me. There wasn't enough time for me to grab my son and leave, so I quickly looked for something I could use as a weapon. The children's playground was free of debris. Without a weapon I decided to move from a sitting position to a standing defensive one. The circumstances determined that I was trapped, outnumbered, and facing a deadly weapon. I recall not feeling panicked. Instead, I just accepting the fact that I was in big trouble and about to get hurt. Then something miraculous happened. Out of nowhere, a young man appeared between myself and the "Leader". He held a small knife in his hand and confronted the man and said "If you want to fight someone, why don't you fight me". The "Leader" immediately said "I don't want any trouble", then he and his gang walked away in the opposite direction.

I thanked my rescuer; got my son and left. I didn't know the person who saved me from this dangerous encounter and never saw him again. Tai Chi Chuan is translated in western vernacular as "The Fist of God". It was God's fist that interceded in the situation and defended me, not my own. The Tai Chi Classics often refers to Divine Intervention.

***

It was a cloudy day in 1980. I was teaching Art at an Alternative High School. Another teacher who I was friends with, stopped in the Art room to borrow art supplies. We were standing next to each other, side by side. For no apparent reason, a visible blue streak of electricity about 8 inches long, shot out from my elbow to her elbow. Along with several students, we both saw and felt it happen. Everyone was amazed. Fa Chin energy is a form of Chi that can be discharged from the body. Also, around this time I was constantly receiving strong static jolts when touching metallic objects, such as doorknobs. During this period, I was heavily involved in the martial arts application of Tai Chi. It was a stage in which I was more focused on projecting Chi in the form of Fa Chin, then storing it as Shen. These visual and tactile experiences involving electrical shocks, made me a firm believer in the power and presence of Chi.

***

In 1982, I was walking in the park with my wife and 8-year-old son. My wife was on my right side. We were talking and holding hands. My son was on my left side and tagging closely along. Over to our far left, about 40 yards away, a group of people were playing soft ball. I heard the crack of a bat hitting a ball and immediately felt a sting in my left hand. When I looked down, I had caught the ball in my bare left hand without being aware of how it happened. More miraculously, the back of my hand holding the softball, was touching my son's nose. If my hand had not caught the ball, it would have done serious damage to my son's face. This is a perfect example of stored Chi performing an action without any conscious effort. I attributed this physical unconscious reaction to the Tai Chi theory that practice will enable your body to make quick and defensive moves without premeditated thought.

***

Around the winter of 1985, I was leaving my parent's home after a Sunday dinner with an armful of leftovers. A mixture of rain and snow had frozen on the 5 concrete steps that lead down to the driveway. When I put my foot down on the top step, both feet slid on the black ice and I went feet first down the steps. Half way down, I landed on my buttocks. Without any conscious or physical effort, I bounced back up and landed on my feet in the driveway. Amazingly enough, I was still holding the left overs in both hands. Chi energy can be manifested as "Jin" or bounce energy. It is a force that can causes things to bounce away from you. I vividly recall the feeling of a soft touch and not the ice-cold hardness of concrete steps. My mother who witness the fall, said she thought I was going to be seriously injured until she saw me bounce back up as if I were on a trampoline.

***

One of the most significant benefit of Tai Chi is its ability to help prolong a healthy life, due to its rejuvenating power. When martial training and applications are not a priority, the Shen Chi that is generated from frequent practiced can be applied towards aiding the recuperating process associated with one's body. My health was excellent until I enter my sixties, then maintenance problems started to arise. Following are cases of how Tai Chi helped me recover from several threatening medical issues.

***

In 2001 I was diagnosed with Bladder Cancer. After surgery, chemo- therapy, and follow-up testing, I asked my Urologist if it was in remission. He said "No it isn't in remission; it is completely gone". One of the intentions of Tai Chi is to rejuvenate the body and prolong good health.

***

In 2006, I had a stroke that was the result of a blocked Vertebral artery. I temporarily lost the peripheral vision in my right eye. A few weeks later, my vision corrected itself and my Neurologist said there were no longer any apparent signs that I had ever had a stroke. The Tai Chi Classics explain how Shen Chi will seek out where the body has been damaged and help make the repair.

***

At the age of 72 in 2017, I had open heart surgery to replace an Aortic valve and a double coronary bypass. Immediately after the operation, family members said they were amazed how well I looked for just coming out of an intensive five-hour, life-threatening surgery. During my hospital stay, the Doctor, Nurses, and Physical Therapist all commented on how quickly I was recovering. Weeks after the procedure, I mentioned to my Primary Physician that I was a little frustrated with so many medical issues after a life time of healthy habits. First, he reiterated the significant influence of hereditary factors. Then, he went on to say that my recuperative ability over the years has been quite remarkable for a man in my age bracket. Furthermore, he found it impressive that my medical issues didn't seem to have a negative impact on my overall quality of life.

***

I contribute my body's ability to regenerate itself to several factors associated with a healthy life style. Surprisingly enough, these same factors can be found in the teachings of the Tai Chi Classics. In Tai Chi, the theory is to help people attain longevity and rejuvenation (Yang L. C. 18th Century AD).

***

I have not been involved in a physical altercation for over 50 years. However, like everyone else, I must defend myself constantly from the trials and tribulations of everyday living. Learning to put my faith in a Divine power stronger than myself has become a natural response for dealing with an array of situations, especially those that I have little or no control of.

***

Spiritual growth is one of the most paramount benefits I have received from the study of Tai Chi. Functioning from a spiritual perspective has proven to be an effective way for dealing with many of the issues that daily existence constantly challenges us with. Tai Chi has been a significant catalyst in providing the necessary insights and spiritual nourishment for living a more rewarding and enriched life.

***

The greatest application of Chi for the whole body is to raise spiritual consciousness (Yang B.H. 19th Century AD).

***

ABOUT THE AUTHOR

The author, Dr. Frank Bisceglia, EdD. has devoted nearly 70 years of his life towards maintaining a healthy level of physical fitness through sports training, exercise and diet. It started with Midget Football then lead to being an All-City Football player at Westinghouse High School. In 1963 he received an Athletic Scholarship to Edinboro University, where he lettered in Football and Wrestling and later coached both sports at Plum Boro High School. He went on to study Yoga, Karate, Kung Fu, and Tai Chi Chuan.

***

Dr. Bisceglia has taught Tai Chi since 1978 for the Y.M.C.A., Community College of Allegheny County, Community College of Beaver County, the Selma Burke Art Center, the Yoga and Meditation Center of Pittsburgh, Unity Center, and the Black Dragon Karate School of Pittsburgh. Over the past 40 years he has taught private lessons and conducted numerous workshops in the surrounding area.

***

In 1969, he got his first exposure to the martial arts while teaching High School Art in Okinawa. In the early 70's, he continued his studies of Shotokan Karate and Kung Fu. He became a student of Tai Chi Chuan in 1975. Along with past visits to South Korea, China and Tibet, he has traveled the world extensively. In 2019 he studied at the Chinese Tai Chi Institute in Taiwan. Dr. Bisceglia has learned different styles of Tai Chi and has been the student of several Tai Chi Masters. However, he has adhered to teaching the traditional Yang style taught by his first instructor and longtime friend, Master Kim Yo-Chou.

***

He earned a B.S. in Art Education in 1967, a Masters in Instructional Design and Technology in 1985, and a Doctorate in Educational Administration in1990. He also studied at the Pittsburgh Theological Seminary.

***

He has taught Art at all levels from preschool to Community College, and retired as an Art Instructor from the Pittsburgh Public School District. He currently teaches Painting at the Community College of Beaver County.

***

REFFERENCES

Basho, M., 16th Century AD. (D. Schiller (ed.). (1994). THE LITTLE ZEN COMPANION. New York, NY: Workman Publishing.

Buddha, 4th Century BC. (T. Byrom (ed.). (1993). DHAMMAPADA: The Sayings of the Buddha. Boston & London. Shabhala Publications, Inc.

Chang, S.-F., 12th Century. Tai Chi Classics I: Treatise. (In L. Waysun (ed.) 1990). *T'AI CHI CLASSICS.* (pp.87-97) Boston, Massachusetts: Shambhala Publications, Inc.

Cheng, M.-C., (1981). TAI CHI CH'UAN: A Simplified Method of Calisthenics for Health & Self Defense. Berkeley, California: North Atlantic Books.

Cheng, M.-C., (1994). T'AI-CHI: The "Supreme Ultimate" Exercise for Health, Sport, and Self-Defense. Rutland, Vermont: Charles E. Tuttle Co.

Cheng, M.-C., (1999). MASTER CHENG'S NEW METHOD of TAI CHI CH'UAN SELF-CULTIVATION. Berkeley, California: Frog, LTD.

Cheng, M.-C., (1985). CHENG TZU'S THIRTEEN TREATISES on T'AI CHI CH'UAN. Berkeley, California: North Atlantic Books.

Chuang, T., 4th Century BC. (L. Kohn (tr.). (2011). THE TAO OF PERFECT HAPPINESS: Selections Annotated & Explained. Woodstock, Vermont: Skylight Paths Publishing.

Dong, Z.-S., 1st Century BC. (L. Waysun (tr.). (1990). TAI CHI CLASSICS. Boston, Massachusetts: Shambhala Publications, Inc.

Einstein, A., 20th Century AD. (D. Schiller (ed.). (1994). THE LITTLE ZEN COMPANION. (p.300). New York, NY: Workman Publishing.

Hui, S., 3rd Century BC. (L. Waysun. (tr.). (1990). TAI CHI CLASSICS. Boston, Massachusetts: Shambhala Publications, Inc.

I CHING, 9TH Century BC. (T. Cleary (tr.). (2017). *I CHING: The Book of Change.* Boulder, Colorado: Shambhala Publications, Inc.

Lao Tzu, 5th Century BC. (J. McDonald (tr.). (2017). TAO TE CHING. Bickels, London: Sirius Publishing.

Lee, B., (1975). TAO OF JEET KUNE DO. Burbank, CA: Ohara Publications, Incorporated.

Li, I.-Y., (19th Century AD). Essentials of the Practice of Form and Push Hands. In B. Lo & M. Inn & R. Amacker & S. Foe. (Ed.) (1985). *THE ESSENCE OF T'AI CHI CH'UAN: The Literary Tradition* (pp.79-82). Berkley, CA: North Atlantic Books.

Li, I.-Y., (19th Century AD). Five Character Secret. In B. Lo & M. Inn & R. Amacker & S. Foe. (Ed.) (1985). *THE ESSENCE OF T'AI CHI CH'UAN: The Literary Tradition* (p.71). Berkley, CA: North Atlantic Books.

Liang, T.T., 21st Century AD. (L. Waysun (tr.). (1990). TAI CHI CLASSICS. Boston, Massachusetts: Shambhala Publications, Inc.

Lin, D., (1964). TAO TE CHING: Annotated & Explained. Woodstock, VT: SkyLight Paths Publishing.

Olson, S. A., (2001). T'AI CHI ACCORDING TO THE I CHING. Rochester, Vermont: Inner Traditions.

Shaw, S., (2002). NIRVANA IN A NUT SHELL. New York, NY. Barnes & Noble Books.

Soong, J.-J., (1995). THE I CHIEN T'AI CHI CH'UAN: With the I Ching Definition of T'ai Chi Ch'uan. Taipei, Taiwan: Chinese Tai Chi Institute.

Song of The Thirteen Postures. (n.d.). In Wen, S.-H. (Ed.) (1973). *FUNDAMNETALS OF TAI CHI CH'UAN* (pp. 409-410). Hong Kong: South Sky book Company.

Suzuki, S., 20th Century AD. (D. Schiller (ed.). (1994). THE LITTLE ZEN COMPANION. (p.1). New York, NY: Workman Publishing.

Tchoung, T.-T., 21st Century AD. (L. Waysun (tr.). 1990). TAI CHI CLASSICS. Boston, Massachusetts: Shambhala Publications, Inc.

Tennant, J., (2010). HEALING IS VOLTAGE: The Hand Book. Scotts Valley. CA: CreateSpace Independent Publishing.

The Eight Truths of Tai Chi. (n.d.). (L. Waysun (tr.). (1990). *TAI CHI CLASSICS*. (pp. 126). Boston, Massachusetts: Shambhala Publications, Inc.

THE LIVING BIBLE. (1972). Edited by Campus Life Magazine. Wheaton, Illinois: Tyndale House Publishers.

Tung, Y.-C., 20th Century AD. (L. Waysun (tr.). (1990). TAI CHI CLASSICS. Boston, Massachusetts: Shambhala Publications, Inc.

Wang T.-Y., 15th Century AD. T'ai Chi Ch'uan Lun. In B. Lo & M. Inn & R. Amacker & S. Foe. (Ed.). (1985). *THE ESSENCE OF T'AI CHI CH'UAN: The Literary Tradition* (pp.29-40). Berkley, CA: North Atlantic Books.

Waysun, L. (1990). TAI CHI CLASSICS. Boston, Massachusetts: Shambhala Publications, Inc.

Wen, S.-H., (1973). FUNDAMENTALS of TAI CHI CH'UAN. Hong Kong: South Sky Book Company.

Wong, C.-Y., 16th Century AD. (L. Waysun (tr.). (1990). TAI CHI CLASSICS. Boston, Massachusetts: Shambhala Publications, Inc.

Wu, Y.-H., 19th Century AD. (L. Waysun (tr.). 1990). TAI CHI CLASSICS. Boston, Massachusetts: Shambhala Publications, Inc

Wu, Y.-H., 19th Century AD. Expositions of Insights into the Practice of the Thirteen Postures. In B. Lo & M. Inn & R. Amacker & S. Foe. (ed.). (1985). *THE ESSENCE OF T'AI CHI CH'UAN: The Literary Tradition* (pp.41-59). Berkley, CA: North Atlantic Books.

Yang, B.- H., 19th Century AD. (L. Waysun (tr.). 1990). TAI CHI CLASSICS. Boston, Massachusetts: Shambhala Publications, Inc.

Yang, C.- F., 20th Century AD. (L. Swaim (tr.). (2005). THE ESSENCE AND APPLICATION OF TAIJIQUAN. Berkeley, California: North Atlantic Books.

Yang, L.-C., 18th Century AD. (L. Waysun (tr.). (1990). TAI CHI CLASSICS. Boston, Massachusetts: Shambhala Publications, Inc.

Yang, Z.-D., 21st Century AD. (L. Waysun (tr.). (1990). TAI CHI CLASSICS. Boston, Massachusetts: Shambhala Publications, Inc.

NOTES / IDEAS

NOTES / IDEAS

.

NOTES / IDEAS

www.ingramcontent.com/pod-product-compliance
Lightning Source LLC
Chambersburg PA
CBHW061403250726
48657CB00004B/1639